I0118744

Yoga of Purification and Transformation

By
Rudra Shivananda

Alight Publications
2004

Yoga of Purification and Transformation

By Rudra Shivananda

First Edition Published in August, 2004

Alight Publications
PO Box 930
Union City, CA 94587

http://www.alightbooks.com

ISBN 1-931833-10-9

Library of Congress Control Number: 2004112274

Printed in the United States of America

Dedicated
to the
Divine Teacher
in all of us
The Inner Guide
who
Lights the Way
and Comforts us
When we Stray

Contents

Introduction

In order to achieve Self-Realization on the path of Yoga, it is absolutely necessary to practice the self-restraints called *yama* which form the first limb of the eightfold (*ashtanga*) path of Yoga as outlined by Patanjali, the expositor of the Yoga Sutras, an authoritative text for all aspiring *yogis*.

When I first started on the spiritual path, I studied the first two limbs of Yoga – *yama* (self-restraint) and *niyama* (self-discipline), and promptly put them aside as "nice" moral or ethical injunctions to which all sane people should subscribe, but really not very "deep" or useful in the practical spiritual techniques to which I was drawn. I very much wanted to start practicing advanced techniques as quickly as possible – a spiritual practice or *sadhana* for Self-Realization.

Most books on Yoga devote a few obligatory pages to these restraints and observances, but seldom lay much stress on their importance or the methods of practice. It is a wonder that hundreds of books have been written on *asana*, the third of the eight limbs, to which Patanjali has given us three verses or sutras, while hardly any books have been written about *yama-niyama*, on which he has written over sixteen sutras!

It has taken me many years to appreciate the importance of *yama-niyama* for speeding up the spiritual journey. Without their practice, the aspiring *yogi* becomes lost in the convoluted jungle of the mind. The *yama-niyama* limbs act as a compass to show the way out of the jungle and towards the goal of liberation.

In these days of fast food and instant gratification, it is indeed difficult for us to imagine that the ancient Masters of Yoga did not instruct a student until the student had prepared and achieved some proficiency by practicing the self-restraints and self-discipline of *yama-niyama*. Even after such preparation, the Master would still demand to observe them for sometime:

To them the Master said, "Stay here for yet another year with austerity, self-control and faith; then you may ask as you please your questions; and if I know then I will surely explain everything to you."
Prasnopanisad 2

Imagine if this happened today! Such a teacher would have very few students, if any. In their compassion the Masters of Yoga nowadays work with students not fully prepared, a much more arduous procedure. There is no culture either in the East or in the West, that now helps to prepare the aspirant in this time of transition. Society seems to reward scoundrels and ethics is considered old-fashioned.

However, let me assure you that there is nothing old-fashioned or unnecessary about the practice of *yama-niyama*. Humanity has not grown out of the necessity for self-restraint and self-discipline. Our very birth in this world is a strong indicator and reminder to us that we are bound by the law of *karma*. This impersonal cosmic law of causation is the means by which we've become propelled from birth to birth – propelled by the cumulative results of each and every action from all our lives. We must face the consequences of all our choices and actions. Our *karmic* predispositions limit and obstruct our path towards Self-Realization. The practice of Yoga removes the obstructions. The practice of the first limb – the five self-restraints of nonviolence, non-lying, non-stealing, non-wastage of energy, and non-attachment enable the aspiring *yogi* to **stop the accumulation of new *karmic* debt**. Without this stoppage of "new *karma*" the practice of the other limbs would be like walking three steps forward and then two and half steps back. The practice of *yama* is the path of purification.

After purification is attained to some degree, the aspiring yogi is ready to remove the blockages caused by nascent *karma*. Ignorance - taking what is unreal as real and what is impermanent as permanent

3

- is one such blockage. The practice of *niyama* – purity, contentment, austerity, self-study and surrender to the Divine – transforms the natural inborn tendencies, turning them on their heads and reverses the flow from involution to evolution, that is the spiritual evolution of the consciousness.

When I explain the practical purposes of *yama-niyama*, most students are surprised but quickly realize how obvious they are. Self-restraint and self-discipline become quickly integrated into their *sadhana*, with remarkable effects of calmness and tranquility.

In the first part of the book I've given a brief overview of each of the five *yama* and five *niyama*. An explanation of *karma* and *dharma*, two cosmic mechanisms, closely associated with *yama-niyama* is given. Since their practice is life-long and life-changing, one of the ways to understand them better is to study the lives of the great *yogis* and sages. The lives of Buddha, Francis of Assisi, Nanak, Gandhi and Martin Luther King are highlighted in the second section for exemplary and inspirational purposes.

In the third section, I've introduced some techniques which enhance our practice of the *yama-niyama*. There is also a more extensive discussion of each of five self-restraints and five self-disciplines. Finally, I conclude in the fourth section, by digging deeper into related dimensions, such as whether *yama* can be absolutely applied without regard to circumstances or whether there should be a relative hierarchy of application, or consideration given to the circumstances.

It is my sincere hope that this work will stimulate greater understanding of the roles of *yama-niyama* in Yoga. I trust that together with the appreciation of their roles, there will be a commitment to adopt them into every spiritual practice. This can only be to the benefit of all sincere practitioners, who are yearning for Self-Realization.

Part 1
Getting Started
Stepping on the path of purification and transformation

The Source of Prosperity

In Ancient India, there was a rich and powerful king who was never satisfied with his lands and wealth. He was especially jealous of his cousins, whom he'd plotted against many times. The eldest cousin was an upright and noble king, who always managed to regain his prosperity, despite all the subterfuges.

The jealous king went to his aged and blind father to learn from him the explanation on how the noble king always came out on top. The father instructed his son by telling him the following story:

There were incessant wars between the forces of light, led by the hero-god Indra and the forces of darkness led by various demon kings. At one time, the demon king was Prahlada, who had transformed his nature to such an extent that he was able to annex the domains of the gods and men by the force of his character and made himself Lord of the three worlds.

Dispossessed, but undaunted, Indra went to the high priest of the gods, Brihaspati, and with all humility, begged him to teach him the means by which he could re-gain his spiritual leadership. Brihaspati taught him the means and said that if he practiced steadfastly it would lead him eventually to paramount virtue.

Indra then asked how that path leading him to spiritual and moral character could be shortened, and Brihaspati counseled him to go learn from the teacher of all the demons. However when the king of light approached the teacher of all the demons, he was in turn counseled to learn directly from his nemesis Prahlada.

Putting on the guise of a spiritual seeker, Indra approached Prahlada and begged him to teach him the path to prosperity. However

Prahlada was fully occupied with the administration all the three worlds and told the disguised Indra that he had no time to take a student. In response Indra fell down at the feet of Prahlada and pleaded that he would wait as long as necessary for instruction from such supreme preceptor.

Pleased with such earnestness, Prahlada chose an auspicious hour to begin, proceeded to teach the highest wisdom to his student, the hero-god. After receiving the teaching in reverence and humility, Indra inquired of Prahlada how he had obtained lordship of the three worlds.

Prahlada replied, "I am never proud that I am king; I do not treat the learned and holy ones with derision. Listening to their words of wisdom I discipline myself and give liberally. They speak to me in confidence and I let myself be guided by them in all things. The sages establish me safely and securely in *dharma* as the bees confine honey in the honeycomb. I have conquered anger and my senses are under my control. In this way I live in the company of those whose speech keeps pace with their understanding, delighting in the light of knowledge. The words of wisdom coming from the lips of a learned person – that is the basis of all prosperity."

After some time had passed, pleased with his student's service and attention, Prahlada offered him a boon and asked him to request whatever he wanted. Whereupon Indra said, "if you are pleased with me and would give me anything I ask for, I would ask for the gift of your character. Please give me your moral character."

Naturally, Prahlada was taken aback by this request and was quite beside himself for a while. Yet a promise is a promise and a boon granted could not be revoked by a noble person. He therefore regretfully made a gift of his entire moral character to the disguised Indra who immediately thanked him and left.

Prahlada was sitting and thinking about what had happened when a spirit of great luster emanated from his body and in response to his startled question said, "I am your moral character and you have divested yourself of me and so I'm going to reside in your student." It then disappeared into the body of Indra.

No sooner had this spirit disappeared, and another great light arose from Prahlada and said, "I am *dharma* and I'm going to your student because I can only reside where there is moral character. Then a third spirit came out of Prahlada's body, even brighter than the previous two and declared himself to be the spirit of truth or *satya* who goes where *dharma* goes.

Immediately after the departure of *satya*, the spirit of good conduct *vritta* rose up together with the spirit of strength, and both left, because strength and good conduct are inseparable.

To make matters worse, a lustrous woman of great divinity appeared and prepared to leave. Prahlada tried to stop her, but she responded, "I am everything that makes for whatever it is auspicious and for prosperity, and I must follow the strength and valor which has left you."

Prahlada realized how his pride and rashness had deprived him of his high moral character. This humbled him and he completely surrendered himself to the Absolute Divine, from whom he had received everything, and to whom he had been so devoted in his childhood.

And so this is how the Lord of the gods, Indra recovered lordship of the three worlds, by learning the secret of moral character from Prahlada. This secret is, "in thought, word and deed, one should refrain from harming any creature. Compassion and giving are the marks of good character. One should not do what may injure another or whatever one would feel ashamed of. Do only that which evokes approval in the assembly of sages. This is the sum and essence of moral character. Even though some people may appear to be prosperous in the world who are not strong in moral character, their prosperity will not last long for its roots are neither deep nor strong. Therefore acquire the virtue of moral character if you wish to attain to lasting prosperity."

Unfortunately, the jealous king did not listen to his father and left unsatisfied. Soon after, he forced a great war against his cousins, but even though he had much larger forces, he was totally destroyed by the upright king.

Karma

It is important for all spiritual aspirants to realize that the practice of self-restraint in the development of moral character is critical to achieving the goal of self-realization. Self-restraint is not merely a set of rules given by religious prophets or social reformers to control the masses, nor is it some ideal philosophical concept. In spiritual practice, self-restraint is the principal path to overcome the spiritual Law of *Karma*.

This spiritual law is the mechanism which impels the soul to re-incarnate and determines the condition, pre-disposition, genetic code etc. of the new birth, based on the actions of the present and past births.

Karma is one of the most important principles in the *Sanatana Dharma*, or ever-present spiritual science of India. The word *karma* has numerous meanings, among them:
- any act or deed
- the principle of cause and effect
- a consequence or "fruit of action" – *karmaphala* [fruit of action] or *uttarphala* [after effect], which sooner or later returns upon the doer. What we sow, we shall reap in this or future lives. Selfish, hateful acts will bring suffering. Benevolent actions will bring loving reactions.

Karma is a neutral, self-perpetuating law of the inner cosmos, much as gravity is an impersonal law of the outer cosmos. In fact, it has been said that gravity is a small, external expression of the greater Law of *Karma*. The impelling, unseen power of one's own past actions is called *adrishta*.

Shri Yukteswar, the great adept of *Kriya Yoga* has affirmed the role of the Law of *Karma* in our lives:

> *All human ills arise from some transgression of universal*
> *law. The scriptures point out that man must satisfy the*
> *laws of nature, while not discrediting the divine*
> *omnipotence. He should say: 'Lord, I trust in Thee, and*
> *Thou can help me, but I too will do my best to undo any*
> *wrong I have done'. By a number of means – by prayer,*
> *by will power, by yoga meditation, by consultation with*
> *saints, by use of astrological bangles – the adverse effects*
> *of past wrongs can be minimized or nullified.*

The Law of *Karma* acts impersonally, yet we may meaningfully interpret its results as either positive [*punya*] or negative [*papa*] – terms describing actions leading the soul either toward or away from the spiritual goal. A good, kind or helpful action increases the store of *punya*, while a harmful action increases one's store of *papa*.

Karma as action is further graded as: white [*sukla*], black [*krishna*], mixed [*sukla-krishna*], or neither white nor black [*asukla-akrishna*]. The latter term describes the *Karma* of the sage or *jnani*, who, as Rishi Patanjali says, is established in *kaivalya*, freedom from delusion through realization of the Self. Similarly, one's own *karma* must be in a condition of *asukla-akrishna*, stable balance, in order for liberation to be attained. The equivalence of *karma* is called *karmasamya*, and is a state of *karmic* equilibrium or resolution in preparation for *samadhi* at death or during spiritual practice.

Karma as the fruit of action is threefold: *sanchita, parabdha,* and *kriyamana*:
- *Sanchita Karma*: this is the accumulated fruit of all one's actions – the sum of all *Karma*s of this life and past lives
- *Parabda Karma*: those fruit of actions begun; set in motion. That portion of *sanchita karma* that is bearing fruit and shaping the events and conditions of the current life, including the nature of one's bodies, personal tendencies

and associations. This is the portion of one's total Karma which has been chosen to bare fruit in the present life.

* *Kriyamana Karma*: The *karma* being created and added to *sanchita* in this life by one's thoughts, words, and actions or in the inner worlds between lives. While some *Kriyamani Karma*s bear fruit in the current life, others are stored for future births.

Another way to look at *karma* is to divide it into two categories: *arabdha* [begun, undertaken] - this is *karma* that is sprouting and *anarabdha* [not commenced] - this is still dormant or seed *karma*.

Karma is the driving force that brings the soul back again and again into human birth in the evolutionary cycle of transmigration called *samsara*. When all earthly *karma*s are resolved and the Self has been realized, the soul is liberated from rebirth.

Whether one believes in re-incarnation or not, there can be little argument about the law of causality in the physical world, and by extension in the spiritual world. As long as one holds a belief in a higher order of being, in some greater potential for all beings, then there is a need to pay attention to the actions that further the realization of the higher potential, and to avoid those actions which hinder this actualization.

For each of the three kinds of *karma* there is a different method of resolution. Nonattachment to the fruits of action, along with daily rites of worship and strict adherence to the codes of *dharma*, stops the accumulation of *kriyamana* or new *karmic* consequences. *Parabdha Karma* is resolved only through being experienced and lived through, and cannot be bypassed. *Sanchita Karma*, the nascent store of *karmic* consequences is normally inaccessible, and can be burned away only through the grace and initiation [*diksha*] of the spiritual guide, who prescribes spiritual practice [*sadhana*] which generates spiritual heat and fire [*tapas*] for the benefit of the earnest spiritual seeker. Through the sustained *kundalini* heat of this *tapas*, the seeds of *karma*s are fried, and therefore will never sprout in this or future lives.

Shri Yogananda, the greatest exponent of *Kriya Yoga* to the West, has affirmed:

> *Seeds of past karma cannot germinate if they are roasted in the fires of divine wisdom.*
>
> *The iron filings of karma are attracted only where a magnet of the personal ego still exists.*

In the state of Self Realization, all latent *karmic* consequences are dissolved, and no future *karma* can be attached. For those who are pre-disposed to the path of knowledge, this has been affirmed by the foremost *Vedantist* Adi Shankaracharya:

> *When everything is known as the Self, not even an atom is seen as other than the Self.... As soon as knowledge of reality has sprung up, there can be no fruits of past actions to be experienced, owing to the unreality of the body, just as there can be no dream after waking.*

For those who are pre-disposed to the path of devotion, Krishna in Bhagavad Gita [9:30-31] re-assures the ardent devotee:

> *Even he with the worst of Karma who ceaselessly meditates on Me quickly loses the effects of his past bad actions. Becoming a high-souled being, he soon attains perennial peace. Know this for certain: the devotee who puts his trust in Me never perishes.*

The five-fold Self-Restraint that we will be discussing next is the practice enjoined implicitly by *Patanjali* for attaining a state of purification, in which no new *karma* is accumulated during all activities of the present life.

Self-Restraint : the taming of the Mind

Self-Restraint (*Yama*) in *yoga* practice is not only a moral or ethical injunction, as in a religious context, but serves very practical and important functions in enabling the goal of spiritual evolution towards self-realization. By the *yogic* practice of Self-restraint, the practitioner's mind is tamed and becomes a conduit for the unfettered experience of higher consciousness, from the Divine, the True Self. Taming of the mind leads to purity of the mind, and only with a pure mind, can one practice and attain to the state of Yoga:

> *Yoga is the cessation [of identifying with] the fluctuations [arising within] consciousness. Then the seer abides in his own true nature.*
> *Patanjali's Yoga Sutras: 1.2-1.3*

This is also elaborated more from a mental and emotional perspective by divine Krishna to his disciple Arjuna:

> *A person whose mind is unperturbed by sorrow, who does not crave pleasures, and who is free from attachment, fear and anger; such a person is a sage of steady wisdom.*
> *Bhagavad Gita: 2.56*

Patanjali, one of the perfected Masters of Yoga or *Siddhas*, wrote very concisely about the integrated science of Yoga. In his *sutras*, he divided the path of *Raja Yoga* or the "Royal Yoga" into eight limbs, referred to as *Ashtanga Yoga*. In these eight limbs he has given us a template to explore the deeper dimensions of Yoga. They are the both the pathways and the unified goal of self-realization. Just as Yoga "is" both the path or means of self-realization, as well as the unified state of super-consciousness that results from the practice, so these eight limbs or *anga* are not only practices, but also states of accomplishment, or perfection.

It is important not to confuse the eight limbs, with 'steps', which can be practiced consecutively and in isolation. Yoga is integration and wholeness – it is the eight limbs practiced together which constitute yoga. However, it is also important to understand that there is a progressive continuity between these limbs, and it is at best futile and at worst spiritually dangerous to try to practice the upper limbs, without first practicing the lower limbs or at least practicing them at the same time. We will explore further their interconnectedness in a later section.

The eight limbs of Yoga are:

1. *yama*: self-restraints through ethical and moral perspective
2. *niyama*: self-discipline through observation of self-realized behavior
3. *asana*: steady posture
4. *pranayama*: control and expansion of the life-energy through the breath
5. *pratyahara*: mind withdrawal from the senses
6. *dharana*: concentration
7. *dhyana*: meditation
8. *samadhi*: super-consciousness or union with the Divine

It is important to "keep in mind", that meditation without the practice of self-restraint or *yama* would not be considered an effective practice of *Ashtanga Yoga*, or *Kriya Yoga*, which is using the *Ashtanga* model. Merely shifting emphasis from one limb to the other does not make one more essential than the other.

> *The restraints are nonviolence, truthfulness, non-stealing,*
> *chastity, and greedlessness.*
> *Yoga Sutras: 2.30*

Another immortal *Siddha*, Tirumoolar, advises a greater number of restraints:

He does not kill, he does not lie, he does not steal,
Of marked virtue he is; good, meek and just;
He shares his joys, he knows no blemish;
Neither drinks nor lusts.
Tirumundirum: 554

We will focus our attention on the five Self-Restraints mentioned by Patanjali. It is important to understand that the *yamas* are interrelated with one another, and also with the *niyamas*, or disciplined observances. For example, the *niyama* contentment [*santosha*] will protect one from stealing. Besides, meaning 'restraint', *yama* is also the name of the King of Death, which calls to mind that there must be a dying to ignorance, which is the source of egoism, attachment and repulsion.

To help us understand and appreciate the Path of Purification and Transformation, it is necessary that we can broaden our perception and learn that we are not just this body which we can see, touch, taste, smell, and hear. Besides the physical body which we are familiar with, we also possess additional subtle bodies. The particular *yogic* model which I like working with assumes that we all possess five bodies.

In addition to the physical body, which we can experience with our five senses, we also have an energy body, which functions with our energy interfaces and stores our basic life-force. Analogous to the physical body with its blood vessels and organs, the energy body has energy channels called *nadis*, and energy centers called *chakras*. A third body is where we store our emotional patterns and the potential energy which function in this mode of our manifestation. The fourth body is the mental body where our mind functions, and is the storage for our mental patterns and associations, as well as for our mental energies. The fifth body is the causal body which is the seat of our soul and repository of our *karmic* patterns from the cause and effect relationships which we have set into play. When we die, only the causal body survives and can be reincarnated into a new physical body.

There are some yogic systems which give more or less bodies and use slightly different names for them, but the basic underlying agreement is that we have more than just the visible body of flesh and blood, or an amorphous mind that is somehow associated with the brain, and that we need to purify and transform all of them.

The *chakras* or energy centers are not on the physical plane, and cannot be discovered by dissecting the physical body. There are seven major *chakras* that are emphasized in the evolutionary path of Yoga. They exist on the other bodies, and their locations can be correlated with various places on our physical body, which is useful for visualization purposes. These *chakras* vibrate at different rates and have an optimum relationship with each other. When they become out of synchronization with each other or with the Universal Life force, then disease of the body and mind can occur.

Situated in the 1st energy center or *Muladahara Chakra*, is the massive potential or nascent life-force energy called *kundalini*, which plays an important role in the process of Self Realization and achievement of higher states of consciousness. Normally, the life-force energy that is available to the energy body is called *prana*. This *prana* is expended during our daily activities and replenished through the air, sun, water, earth and food. Only with intense yogic practice and purification of the physical and subtle bodies will the *kundalini* energy be available.

By practicing the self-restraints, the subtle energy body, with its energy channels are purified, enabling more energy and life-force to flow through them. This also eases the upward movement of the *kundalini* through the *chakras*. Therefore any kind of *Hatha, Kundalini,* and *Kriya Yogas*, which works directly with life-force energy, whether in the form of *prana* or *kundalini*, must incorporate the practice of the *yamas*.

We are all beset with obstacles and problems as we turn towards the divine, to reach our highest potential. It is necessary to be constantly examining your thoughts, words and actions with awareness and discrimination - you will then come to an understanding of why problems and obstacles occur, and by which means they can be avoided. By turning the attention within (Self-awareness) to observe the inner obstacles, thoughts and feelings, the obstructions will be revealed. You will realize what agitates the mind and veils the truth. The *yamas* are to be practiced in thought, word and deed, for example, negative thoughts, harsh words, and physical hurt are all lack of restraint of nonviolence or *ahimsa*.

The Path of Purification
Yama

Ahimsa (nonviolence)**,** *satya* (truthfulness)**,**
asteya (non-stealing)**,** *brahmacharya* (self-control)**, and**
aparigraha (non-attachment) are the five restraints.
Yoga Sutras 2:30

Ahimsa (**nonviolence**): To refrain from causing pain to any living being, including oneself. Every action, word, or thought that causes pain to another - any thought containing anger, hatred, greed, lust, or attachment - is a form of violence. With the perfection of *ahimsa*, one's nonviolent nature and peace radiate to others. Even violent creatures (e.g. wild animals) abandon their hostility in the presence of such a non-violent being.

Satya (**truthfulness**): To develop honesty; to avoid deceiving others and oneself. Cultivating truthfulness requires the aspirant to avoid exaggeration, rationalization, pretense, and all other variations of deceit. When truthfulness is perfected, one's words and blessings always come true. The highest form of *satya* is discovery of one's true nature.

Asteya (**non-stealing**): To avoid any kind of misappropriation of material or non-material things, for example, even acceptance of undeserved praise can be *asteya*. When non-stealing is perfected, one is freed from the illusion of ownership: me/mine, you/yours.

Brahmacharya (**self-control**): To conserve and redirect the all forms of energy, especially sexual energy. Literally translated, *brahmacharya* means "to walk on God's path". Perfect celibacy is, above all, an attitude of mind - purity of thought, word, and deed. To aid in the practice of celibacy one should eat *sattvic* food and avoid worldly situations and environments. When continence is perfected, one gains physical, mental, and spiritual strength.

Aparigraha (**non-attachment**): To avoid the accumulation of unnecessary possessions. Its purpose is to become free not from possessions themselves, but attachment to them so that one is unaffected by their gain or loss. Perfection of *aparigraha* gives dispassion and one gains knowledge of the past, present, and future.

Suggested practice:

Examine each of the five restraints in turn. Think about what they mean to you. Write out 2-3 pages on each. This will help you to put them into perspective, as you learn more about them in the later parts of the book.

Before going to bed in the night, sit for about 5 minutes in a quiet place and observe your thoughts, words and deeds, how they may relate to the five restraints. This will help you to move into a state of self-awareness and mindfulness that is essential for the practice of the restraints.

Dharma

It is not enough that the spiritual practitioner is purified by the practice of self-restraint. The eradication of the *karmic* storehouse or *sanchita karma* requires perfection in *dharma*.

The word *dharma* is from *dhri* – to sustain, carry, hold – that which contains or upholds the cosmos. It is a complex, all-inclusive term with many meanings, including: divine law, law of being, way of righteousness, religion, duty, responsibility, virtue, justice, goodness and truth.

Essentially, *dharma* is the orderly fulfillment of an inherent nature or destiny – each of us has his or her *dharma* – the best path to self-realization. Relating to the soul, it is the mode of conduct most conducive to spiritual advancement, the right and righteous path.

There are four principal kinds of *dharma*:

- *Rita* : universal law - the inherent order of the universe. The law of being and nature that contain and govern all forms, functions and processes, from galaxy clusters to the power of mental thought and perception. This is also the foundation of all physical and scientific laws.
- *Varna dharma*: social duty – law of one's own kind. This defines an individual's obligations and responsibilities within the nation, society, community, class, occupational subgroup and family. An important part of this *dharma* is religious moral law.
- *Asrama dharma*: duties of life's stages. Human *dharma*. The natural process of maturing from childhood to old age through fulfillment of the duties of each of the four stages of life – *brahmachari* (student), *grihasta* (householder), *vanaprastha* (elder advisor), and *sannyasa* (religious

recluse) – in pursuit of the four human goal : *dharma* (righteousness), *artha* (wealth), *kama* (pleasure) and *moksha* (liberation).

* S*vadharma*: personal law – one's perfect individual pattern through life, according to one's own particular physical, mental and emotional nature. S*vadharma* is determined by the sum of past *Karma*s and the cumulative effect of the other three *dharma*s. It is the individualized application of *dharma*, dependent on personal *Karma*, reflected on one's race, community, physical characteristics, health, intelligence, skills and aptitudes, desires and tendencies, religion, *sampradaya* [spiritual lineage], family and *guru*.

A part of the social duty of each person is called the principle of good conduct that applicable to all people regardless of age, gender or class. It is listed in the ancient *Manu Sastras* as : steadfastness, forgiveness, self-restraint, non-stealing, cleanliness, sense control, high-mindedness, learning, truthfulness, absence of anger. These are also called *samanya dharma* – the general duty of all beings.

The ancients were wise enough to provide for exceptions to the general rules, and called it *apad dharma* or emergency conduct, for which the only rigid rule is wisdom. Exceptional situations may require deviating from normal rules of conduct, with the condition that such exceptions are to be made only for the sakes of others, not for personal advantage.

Thoughts, words or deeds that transgress divine law in any of the human expressions of *dharma* is unrighteousness and is called *adharma*. They bring the accumulation of demerits called *papa*, while *dharma* brings merit, called *punya*.

It is by the practice of *niyama* or the self discipline of observances that the spiritual seeker is transformed into a perfected being who is the essence of *dharma*.

Through the active practice [*tapas*] and self-study [*svadyaya*], the *yogi* becomes united with *dharma*. It is said that if one knows and acts according to one's dharma, then one is pure [*saucha*], content [*santosha*], and surrendered to the divine will [*ishvar pranidhana*].

Self Discipline: Transforming the Soul

While *yama* purifies the mind, we must understand *yogic* physiology
to place the mind in proper perspective. The mind or *manas* is a
mode of the mental body, used effectively for dealing with the world
of the five senses, and as such is a barrier to higher consciousness.
Manas is a fine tool for what it is meant to do, but because of the
dominance of another mode called "I-ness" or *ahamkara*, it has
malfunctioned and can no longer provide an accurate representation
of the world.

Ahamkara which serves the function of a temporary separation of
identity is useful in experiencing limitation for an unlimited
consciousness. However, when *ahamkara* is dominant, there is a
loss of the connection to the unlimited consciousness, and the mind
or *manas* can only experience the world in an egocentric miasma
of confusion, doubt and fear. The sensory images from *manas* are
filtered through *ahamkara*, resulting in likes and dislikes,
possessiveness, and desires. Through the conscientious practice
of the five self-restraints of *yama*, the grip of "I-ness" is dislodged
and *manas* is freed to experience the world as it is.

The spiritual seeker first must begin the practice of the self-restraints
and remove the barrier of the mind before Self-realization can be
achieved. However, the aspiring *yogi* need not wait to begin
practice of the five-fold self-discipline of the *niyama*.

There is a higher mode of consciousness beyond the mind and the
"I-ness". It is called *buddhi* or "light of wisdom" or the "clear
mind of pure consciousness". There is no good English translation
for *buddhi*, and the normal one used is intellect which is inadequate,
as is discriminatory mind.

The self-discipline of *niyama* lets the light of *buddhi* shine through
the purified *manas*, such that the spiritual aspirant begins to see

reality as it is. As the *buddhi* brings light to the darkness of ignorance, the practice of *yama* is perfected and requires less and less effort until it becomes effortless.

By the practice of purifying the body and mind [*saucha*] and cultivating contentment [*santosha*], one is able to loosen the hold of the ego. Then through the practice of self-study [*svadyaya*] and surrender to the Divine [*ishvar pranidhana*], the light of *buddhi* is allowed to shine forth and illuminate the seeker's life.

The Path of Transformation
Niyama

Shaucha (purity), *santosha* (contentment), *tapas* (austerity),
svadyaya (self- study), and *Ishvarapranidhana* (surrender to
Divine) constitute observances.
Yoga Sutras 2:32

Shaucha (**purity**): Cleanliness of the body and purity of the mind.
As the mind and body are interdependent, purification of the body
is a means of controlling the mind...

By observing cleanliness one becomes less attached to one's own
body. When purity is perfected one gains control of the senses and
becomes cheerful, one-pointed, and fit for Self-realization.

Santosha (**contentment**): not just a passive state of mind,
contentment is a virtue to be actively cultivated in order to free the
mind from the effects of pleasure and pain. When contentment is
perfected, one becomes desire-less and attains unexcelled happiness.

Tapas (**austerity**): Literally, "to burn"; in Yoga *tapas* implies the
burning of all desires by means of discipline, purification, and
penance. Fasting, enduring heat or cold, and observing silence are
examples of gross methods of *tapas*. Any form of giving up desires
is *tapas*. *Pranayama* (breath expansion and control) is considered
to be the highest austerity, as it requires great restraint of the normal,
life-giving breath. When austerity is perfected one achieves control
over the body and the senses. In a sense all techniques of Yoga can
be considered as forms of *tapas*.

Svadhyaya (self-study): This includes all Self-inquiry, study of
scriptures, *satsang* (spiritual meetings), and *japa* (repetition) of
Om, with the aim of attaining liberation. Studying the inspirational
and holy literature, as well as studying the lives and teachings of

saints is helpful in the beginning. Self-inquiry is done by reflecting deeply on the question, "Who am I?" *Satsang* is association with spiritually oriented people and places. As *Om* is the origin of all *mantras* (sacred sounds or words), the *japa* of *Om* may be extended to include any *mantras* used for liberation. Through *svadhyaya* one can contact the form of the Divine with whom one desires to have a deeper relationship.

Ishvarapranidhana (surrender to Divine): This is the recognition that the limited, ego-self is an illusion and the channeling of energies toward the realization of truth, or the Divine. One who sees the Self in all beings and who has surrendered the ego of being the "doer" is the true practitioner of *Ishvarapranidhana*. Perfection of *Ishvarapranidhana* brings success in *samadhi* or super-consciousness.

Suggested Practice:

Consider each of the *niyama*, and how they may relate to your life at this time. How do you deal with purity of body or mind? Are you pursuing some kind of self-study? Is this something that appeals to you? Is there something pro-active that you can do to increase you level of contentment? Have you been thinking that contentment was a future state that will "happen" after some sort of spiritual epiphany?

.

Part 2
Inspiration and Instruction
from the Lives of
Spiritual Role Models

Siddartha Gautama

The Buddha is "one who is awakened, or enlightened." He is also known as the *Tathagata*, which means "the one who has come thus," and *Shakyamuni*, which means "the sage of the Shakya tribe." He is said to have lived eighty years, and thus was probably born in 563 BCE, as his death in 483 BCE has been historically documented.

The Buddha's birth name was Siddartha, which means "he who has accomplished his aim," and the name of his clan was Gautama. A famous seer named Asita predicted that the child would either become a great king or, if he left home, a great teacher.

Siddhartha was raised amid the finest luxuries of the time. It was said that three palaces had been built for him - one for hot weather, one for cold, and one for the rainy season. As a prince, he was trained in all the martial arts and excelled in all of them, especially archery. When he was about sixteen years old, he chose for his wife the beautiful Yasodhara, and for the next thirteen years he lived the life of the householder with his wife and concubines.

The future Buddha's father had tried to prevent his princely son from experiencing any suffering or sorrow or religious contact so that he would become a king rather than a spiritual teacher. However, one day while traveling outside the palace gates, Siddhartha happened to come across a very old man for the first time in his life. He was appalled at the wrinkles and decrepitude, especially when he learnt from his servant that old age happened to all men. On another occasion he happened to observe a sick person and learned about the loathsome nature of disease. The third sign came when he witnessed a funeral procession and was able to see the lifeless corpse that was being carried. The suddenness of these three experiences set him thinking about the transitory nature of human life. Finally he came upon a religious ascetic, who had renounced the world to seek enlightenment, and marveled at his serenity.

Siddhartha felt that he had fulfilled his obligation to continue his family line when his son Rahul had been born and decided that he too must renounce his kingdom and seek a way out of the human miseries of old age, sickness, and death. In the dark of night he secretly left the palace, throwing off his princely garments and donning the robe of an ascetic. He cut his princely locks and began his journey walking to seek enlightenment.

Following the footsteps of the sages of *Sanatana Dharma*, Siddhartha practiced Yoga and meditation. He studied meditative concentration at the feet of Alara Kalama, a leading Master of the time. The former prince made astonishing progress and when he could reach the formless state, his Guru gave his blessings and sent him on to Uddaka Ramaputra, from whom he then learnt to attain the higher state of consciousness beyond thought and non-thought. After stabilizing at this state, he was given the Guru's blessings and instructed to find his own path to the ultimate and perfect enlightenment.

Siddhartha, the renunciate decided to practice the path of extreme austerities, and in this he was joined by five other *yogis*. For six years they tortured their bodies with extreme techniques but instead of achieving cosmic consciousness and wisdom they only seemed to get weaker and weaker. Finally Siddhartha the ascetic, who was now just a bag of bones decided that there must be a better way to attain enlightenment. He felt that he needed to regain his strength for the concentration needed, and so he decided to start eating again. When he gave up practicing the extreme austerities, the other five ascetics who were with him became disillusioned and left him,

It became clear to Gautama that a life of penance and pain was no better than a life of luxury and pleasure, because if penance on earth is to be the religion, then how could the heavenly reward for penance be bliss? If merit came merely from purity of food, then the deer should have the most merit. One who practices asceticism without calming the passions is like a man trying to kindle fire by rubbing a stick on green wood in water, but one who has no desires or worldly attachments is like a man using a dry stick that ignites.

After he had regained his strength, Siddhartha once again practiced meditation. First he attained the state of joy and pleasure, followed by blissful state arising from concentration with serenity and the mind fixed on one point without reasoning and investigation. The third stage gave rise to equanimity from joy and aversion, followed by the fourth stage in which pleasure and pain were left behind in a mindful purity. When his mind was concentrated and cleansed he directed it to the remembrance of former existences in previous births, piercing the cycles of evolution and dissolution of the universe.

Then he focused on the passing away and rebirth of beings, perceiving how the *karma* of negative actions, words, and thoughts led to rebirth in misery, while those beings leading good lives are reborn in a happy state. Finally his consciousness focused on the means of ultimate release and he realized that the four noble truths – that there is pain, a cause of pain, the cessation of pain, and a way that leads to that cessation of pain. Thus his mind was freed from sensual desires, the desire for existence, and ignorance.

According to legend this whole process occurred in one night after he had decided to sit under a tree until he became enlightened or died. And so by his determination, darkness and ignorance were dispelled with the light, just as Siddhartha Gautama became enlightened and was then known as the Buddha.

The Buddha gave his first sermon in a deer park in *Benares*. He explained that the two extremes are not to be practiced by the one who wishes to be enlightened - passion and luxury which degrades morals, nor painful self-torture which is disguised attachment. Avoiding these two extremes the enlightened follows the middle path which produces insight and knowledge that leads to peace, wisdom, enlightenment, and *nirvana*. Buddha then expounded the four noble or *aryan* truths of his doctrine:

> *Now this, aspirants, is the noble truth of pain:*
> *birth is painful; old age is painful;*
> *sickness is painful; death is painful;*
> *sorrow, lamentation, dejection, and despair are painful.*
> *Contact with unpleasant things is painful;*
> *not getting what one wishes is painful.*
> *In short the five groups of grasping are painful.*
> *Now this is the noble truth of the cause of pain:*
> *the craving, which leads to rebirth,*
> *combined with pleasure and lust,*
> *finding pleasure here and there,*
> *that is the craving for passion,*
> *the craving for existence,*
> *even the craving for non-existence.*
> *Now this is the noble truth of the cessation of pain:*
> *the cessation without a remainder of craving,*
> *abandonment, forsaking, release, and non-attachment.*
> *Now this is the noble truth*
> *of the way that leads to the cessation of pain:*
> *this is the noble eightfold way, namely,*
> *right understanding, right intention,*
> *right speech, right action, right livelihood,*
> *right effort, right concentration,*
> *and right meditation.*

The foundation of spiritual life is well-expressed in his teachings as preserved in the *Dhammapada*: we are the result of our thoughts, so one who is always complaining is full of hatred, while one who forgives is filled with love. The person who uses violence is not just; rather the just person learns and uses intelligence to distinguish right from wrong and to guide others. A good person is tolerant with the intolerant, mild with the violent, and free from greed among the greedy:

> *Everyone trembles at punishment and everyone loves life; remember that you are like them, and do not kill nor cause slaughter. Do not speak harshly to anyone, for angry speech is painful. Let a person overcome anger by love, let him overcome evil by good; let him overcome greed by generosity, and lying by truth.*

Once while the Buddha was out walking with a group of his disciples in a village, all the villagers started to run about in fear. A raging elephant was running loose and trampling all in its path. The disciples started to run away but the Buddha did not move. He stood still, right in its path and sent his love to the elephant, and the rage went out of it. The elephant meekly knelt before the Buddha. Such is the power of perfected nonviolence or *ahimsa* that even wild animals are tamed in its presence.

Buddha taught the law of *karma* and the importance of individual effort. A disciple once asked him why people differed so much in birth, intelligence, health, and so on. The Enlightened One explained that beings are the product of their *karma*, the consequences of their actions. Evildoers may experience happiness until their evil deeds ripen, and the good may experience bad things until their good deeds ripen. The pure and the impure create their own destinies and no one can purify another.

At another time the Buddha and a thousand disciples dwelled near a volcanic mountain with its glowing fire. The Buddha preached his sermon on fire - how the sensations, perceptions, thoughts, and actions are burning with the poisons of covetousness, anger, and ignorance. Only be self-restrain and self-discipline, by following the precepts laid down, can the fire be extinguished.

A skeptic told the Buddha that he could not accept any conclusive doctrine. The Enlightened One simply asked him if he recognized his own doctrine as conclusive. Caught in self-contradiction, the skeptic realized the weakness and limitation of skeptical philosophy, and became a disciple.

The Buddha had a half-brother who was about to be declared crown prince and married to Sundari, the most beautiful woman in the kingdom. Instead he decided to join the community that had gathered around Shakyamuni and become a monk. However, he could not help thinking about the beautiful Sundari, and so to motivate him, the Buddha promised him that if he attained enlightenment he would have hundreds of heavenly damsels, giving him a vision of these even more beautiful maidens. Eventually after attaining a degree of dispassion, he discarded this motivation and asked the Buddha to dissolve his promise of the maidens, and soon after attained enlightenment, becoming an *arhat*, a noble one.

Complaints that monks wandering around during the rainy season trampled the grass and destroyed living creatures led the Buddha to adopt the custom of staying in retreat during the three months of rain.

A new monk once confessed to the Buddha that he had eaten meat in his alms-bowl, but the Buddha forgave him and all those who ate meat that was not prepared for them. The ethical principle was not to harm any living creature, and so he criticized those who hunt and kill animals for sport.

Although many of his disciples became monks, the Buddha declared that a lay disciple, whose mind is free from the poisons of lust, attachment, false views, and ignorance, was no different than anyone else who is free. It was more difficult for a lay person to achieve enlightenment, but once achieved, there was no difference in quality of enlightenment between a monk and a lay follower.

Fearing a famine the warrior chiefs of one tribe decided to battle against another tribe over water rights because the latter had built a dike to conserve water and refused to dismantle it. Just before the battle was to begin, the Buddha spoke to both sides, asking them to compare the value of earth and water to the intrinsic value of people and the human blood they were about to spill. He then told a parable about demon who fed on anger. The demon assumed the guise of a king and took over a royal throne, becoming stronger as more anger was directed at him until the true king came and calmly offered to serve the throne which led to the diminishment and disappearance of the anger demon. The two tribes made peace and in this way the war was avoided.

A woman was stricken with grief when her only son died. Unable to find a physician who could bring him back to life, she went to the Buddha. He told her that before he would bring his son back from the dead, she had to get him a handful of mustard seed in the city, but it must be from a house where no one has ever lost a child, spouse, parent, or friend. Eventually she came to realize how common death was and put aside her selfish attachment to her child.

A monk entreated the Buddha to explain whether the world is eternal or temporary, finite or infinite, whether life and the body are the same or different, whether *arhats* are beyond death or not. First the Buddha pointed out that he had never promised to explain these things. Then he told the parable of a man who had been pierced by a poisoned arrow, and his relatives had summoned a doctor. Suppose the physician had said that he would not remove the arrow or treat the patient until his questions had been answered; such as who made the bow, what kind it was, all about the arrow, and so on. The man would die, and still the information would not be known. Then the Buddha announced that a person would come to the end of his life before those metaphysical questions could be answered by the Enlightened One. Those questions do not tend toward edification nor lead to supreme wisdom. The Buddha's teaching regarding suffering, its cause, and the means of ending it is like removing the poisoned arrow.

When they came to a town and saw animal sacrifices being made to edify the gods, the Buddha advised his followers not to be deceived by such outward acts but to purify their hearts and cease to kill. The only sacrifice accepted by the Divine is a pure body and a calm mind devoted to attaining the qualities of loving friendship, compassion, altruistic joy, and equanimity.

When some noblemen with a low-caste servant came for initiation, the Buddha initiated the servant first, declaring that in regard to the ascetic life, there can be no separation of castes.

A monk proposed to spread Buddha's teachings among a wild and dangerous tribe. Foreseeing what would happen, the Buddha asked him what he would do if they insulted and abused him. The monk answered that he would consider them good and kind for not hitting him and throwing rocks at him. But what if they hit and threw rocks? Then he would be glad they did not use clubs and swords. If they did use clubs and swords, he would be glad they did not kill him, and even if they kill him, they will have delivered him from his body, to a higher existence. So equipped with patience and love, the monk set out and started to teach among these savages. He was about to be killed by an archer just for fun, when the hunter was so struck by his willingness to die that he stopped and eventually the savage tribe became followers.

The Enlightened One was established in the unity of Being. He was able to tame a dangerous robber and admitted him into the community. On another occasion, he bathed and treated a monk, who was suffering from dysentery and had been neglected by the other monks because he lay in his own excrement. He even took a leper as a disciple. When he was 72 years old, his enemies sent hired killers to dispose of him – the compassionate Buddha converted them.

Throughout his life, Shakyamuni taught and showed great forgiveness. Once a king who had persecuted the Buddha's disciples and secretly had his father, a disciple of the Buddha imprisoned and killed, confessed his sin in putting to death his father and asked to be a disciple of the blessed one. The Buddha accepted his confession and noted that in the tradition of the noble ones' discipline, whoever sees one's fault as a fault and correctly confesses it shall attain self-restraint in the future.

When he was about to cast off his body at the age of eighty, and before going through the four stages of higher awareness into *mahanirvana*, the last words of the Buddha were, "Decay is inherent in all component things. Work out your own salvation with diligence."

The Buddha described himself simply:

> *as a binder together of those who are divided,*
> *an encourager of those who are friends,*
> *a peacemaker, a lover of peace, impassioned for peace,*
> *a speaker of words that make for peace.*

The Enlightened One identified the causal chain of suffering in his theory of dependent arising:

> *Sorrow, lamentation, misery, grief, despair, old age, and*
> *death are all caused by birth,*
> *which depends on existence,*
> *which depends on attachment,*
> *which depends on desire,*
> *which depends on sensation,*
> *which depends on contact,*

which depends on the six senses,
which depend on name and form,
which depend on consciousness,
which depends on karma,
which depends on ignorance.
Therefore, by ending ignorance, then karma,
consciousness, name and form, the six senses, contact,
sensation, desire, attachment, existence, and birth with all
the misery that comes after birth can be ended.

He taught that ignorance could be ended by mindfulness and self-restraint. The Buddha always emphasized the importance of mindfulness toward the ethical significance of every action and word. After having mastered the moral precepts, restrained the senses, endowed with mindfulness and self-possession, filled with contentment, the seeker should then choose a lonely and quiet spot to meditate in order to purify the mind of lusts, the wish to injure, ill temper, sloth, worry, irritability, wavering, and doubt.

The five precepts are that the Buddha enjoins us to practice are:

Do not kill any living being.
Do not take what is not given to you.
Do not speak falsely.
Do not drink intoxicating drinks.
Do not be unchaste.

The Buddha's life teaches us the importance of love. In the very first verse of his path of righteousness, he says:

Hate is never conquered by hate.
Hate is conquered by love.
This is an eternal law.

Francis of Assisi

Where there is charity and wisdom,
there is neither fear nor ignorance.
Where there is patience and humility,
there is neither anger nor vexation.
Where there is poverty and joy,
there is neither greed nor avarice.
Where there is peace and meditation,
there is neither anxiety nor doubt.

Francis of Assisi (1182-1226) was the son of a rich cloth merchant. He was born while his father was traveling in France; his mother named him Giovanni, after John the Baptist, but when his father returned he changed his name to Francis, for the country which had infatuated him.

Francis enjoyed a very rich and easy life growing up because of his father's wealth and the permissiveness of the times. He became the leader of a crowd of young people who spent their nights in wild parties. His biographer who knew him well, said, "In other respects an exquisite youth, he attracted to himself a whole retinue of young people addicted to evil and accustomed to vice." Francis said of himself during that time, "I lived in sin."

When he was twenty a neighboring town made war on Assisi, and Francis was imprisoned for a year with some of the nobles from his city. This gave him time to reflect and study the scriptures. However, his mind was still turned towards becoming a knight and winning glory. After his release, Francis went back to his fun-loving ways, until a call for knights for the Fourth Crusade gave him a chance for his dream. He outfitted himself with armor and horse and set out with the support of his father and townspeople.

But Francis never got farther than one day's ride from Assisi. There he had a dream in which God told him he had it all wrong, asking why he would leave the Lord and serve a vassal, telling him to return home. His return was greeted with laughter and humiliation.

The Transformation

Francis started to spend more time in prayer. He went off to a cave and wept for his sins. Sometimes God's grace overwhelmed him with joy.

One day while riding through the countryside, Francis, the man who loved beauty, who was so picky about food, who hated deformity, came face to face with a leper. Repelled by the appearance and the smell of the leper, Francis nevertheless jumped down from his horse and kissed the hand of the leper. When his kiss of peace was returned, Francis was filled with joy. As he rode off, he turned around for a last wave, and saw that the leper had disappeared. He always looked upon it as a test from God...that he had passed.

His search for conversion led him to the ancient church at San Damiano. While he was praying there, he heard Christ on the crucifix speak to him, "Francis, repair my church." Francis assumed this meant the old church building he was in and immediately took fabric from his father's shop and sold it to get money to repair the church. His father was not pleased.

Growing increasingly frustrated with Francis's erratic behavior, his father decided to disown him in public. Francis stripped off all his clothes — the clothes his father had given him — until he was wearing only a shirt, and surrendered himself completely to the providence of the Lord. Wearing nothing but castoff rags, he went off into the freezing woods — singing. Later when robbers beat him and took even his rags, he climbed out of the ditch they had thrown him into and went off singing again. From then on Francis had nothing...and everything.

Slowly companions came to Francis, people who wanted to follow his life of sleeping in the open, begging for garbage to eat...and loving God. With companions, Francis knew he now had to have some kind of direction to his life and so he opened the Bible in three places. He read the command to the rich young man to sell all of his goods and give to the poor, the order to the apostles to take nothing on their journey, and the demand to take up the cross daily. "Here is our rule," Francis said — as simple, and as seemingly impossible, as that. He was going to do what no one thought possible any more — live by the Gospel. Francis took these commands so literally that he made one brother run after the thief who had stolen his hood and offer him his robe!

Francis practiced true equality by showing honor, respect, and love to every person whether they were beggar or pope. Following the teachings of the Christ as closely as possible he and his disciples vowed to live in abject poverty while doing works of charity. Within eleven years there were over five thousand Franciscan Friars. He also founded the Poor Clares for women and later the Third Order for people who lived in the world. The Rules of the Franciscan Order were ratified by Pope Innocent III.

In 1210 through his personal intervention and constant preaching, an agreement was reached between the upper and lower classes of Assisi which foreshadowed the Magna Charta by granting bondsmen the right to free themselves from their lords.

Francis traveled to Egypt in 1212 to preach in a Crusaders' camp, and then in spite of warnings of the danger he entered Saracen territory. When he and his only companion were seized and bound by the Muslim solders, Francis shouted, "Sultan! Sultan!" Brought to the Sultan he shared the message of Christ and challenged a priest of Mohammed to enter the flames with him to see whose faith was stronger. The Sultan was impressed by his courage and gave Francis gold, silver, silk, and precious things, but Francis refused them all. The Sultan let the two friars go free and gave Francis and his followers permission to travel through Saracen lands. Francis was then able to visit Bethlehem, Jerusalem and Mount Calvary.

His Teachings and Stories

But Francis would not let his followers accept any money. They worked for all necessities and only begged if they had to. He told them to treat coins as if they were pebbles in the road. When a bishop showed horror at the friars' hard life, Francis said, "If we had any possessions we should need weapons and laws to defend them." Possessing something was the death of love for Francis. He reasoned - what could you do to a man who owns nothing? You can't starve a fasting man, you can't steal from someone who has no money, you can't ruin someone who hates prestige. Only one who had nothing was truly free.

He even gave up authority in the orders which he had founded, demonstrating that true freedom lies in non-attachment. When Francis became blind and ill, he transcended his suffering by his non-attachment, composing his famous praise of the Divine, the Canticle of the Sun.

The Canticle of Brother Sun

Most High, all-powerful, all-good Lord,
All praise is Yours, all glory,
all honor and all blessings.
To you alone, Most High, do they belong,
and no mortal lips are worthy

to pronounce Your Name.

Praised be You my Lord with all Your creatures,
especially Sir Brother Sun,
Who is the day through whom You give us light.
And he is beautiful and radiant with great splendor,
Of You Most High, he bears the likeness.

Praised be You, my Lord, through Sister Moon
and the stars,
In the heavens you have made them
bright, precious and fair.

Praised be You, my Lord, through
Brothers Wind and Air,
And fair and stormy, all weather's moods,
by which You cherish all that You have made.

Praised be You my Lord through Sister Water,
So useful, humble, precious and pure.

Praised be You my Lord through Brother Fire,
through whom You light the night
and he is beautiful and playful and robust and strong.

Praised be You my Lord through our Sister,
Mother Earth who sustains and governs us,
producing varied fruits with colored flowers and herbs.

Praise be You my Lord through those who grant pardon
for love of You and bear sickness and trial.
Blessed are those who endure in peace,
By You Most High, they will be crowned.

Praised be You, my Lord through Sister Death,

from whom no-one living can escape.
Woe to those who die in mortal sin!
Blessed are they She finds doing Your Will.
No second death can do them harm.

Praise and bless my Lord and give Him thanks,
And serve Him with great humility.

Once Brother Leo asked Francis to describe perfect joy, and Francis related that if, when wet, cold, and muddy, they knocked on a convent door, but the porter refused to let them in and drove them away like a couple of thieves, beating them with clubs until they nearly died, "and if we endure all this so patiently, and think of the sufferings of Christ, the All-praised One, and of how much we ought to suffer for the sake of our love of him - O Brother Leo, mark thou, that in this is perfect joy."

Francis Preaches to the Birds

Francis demonstrated repeatedly that he had perfected *ahimsa* or nonviolence. At one time, Francis and his companions were making a trip through a village when he spotted a great number of birds of all varieties. There were doves, crows and all sorts of birds. Inspired by divine love, Francis left his friends on the road and ran after the birds, who patiently waited for him. He greeted them in his usual way, expecting them to scurry off into the air as he spoke. But they did not move.

With pure mind and intention, he asked them if they would stay awhile and listen to the Word of God. He said to them: "My brother and sister birds, you should praise your Creator and always love him: He gave you feathers for clothes, wings to fly and all other things that you need. It is God who made you noble among all creatures, making your home in thin, pure air. Without sowing or reaping, you receive God's guidance and protection."

At this the birds began to spread their wings, stretch their necks and gaze at Francis, in a wonderful way according to their nature. Francis then walked right through the middle of them, turned around and came back, touching their heads and bodies with his tunic. Then he gave them his blessing, making the sign of the cross over them. At that they flew off and Francis, rejoicing and giving thanks to God, went on his way.

From that day on, Francis made it his habit to solicitously invoke all birds, all animals and reptiles to praise and love their Creator. And many times during Francis' life there were remarkable events of Francis speaking to the animals. There was even a time when he quieted a flock of noisy birds that were interrupting a religious ceremony! Much to the wonder of all present, the birds remained quiet until Francis' sermon was complete.

> *Heavenly Father,*
> *You gave Your servant Francis*
> *great love for each of Your creatures.*
> *Teach us to see Your design in all of creation.*
> *We ask this in Jesus' Name. Amen.*

Francis, Rabbits and Fish

One day when a rabbit that had been caught in a trap was brought to him, Francis advised the rabbit to be more alert in the future, then released the rabbit from the trap and set it on the ground to go its way. But the rabbit hopped back up onto Francis' lap, desiring to be close to the saint.

Francis took the rabbit a few steps into the woods and set it down. But it followed Francis back to his seat and hopped on his lap again! Finally Francis asked one of his fellow friars to take the rabbit far into the woods and let it go. That worked. This type of thing happened repeatedly to Francis - which he saw as an opportunity to praise the glory of God.

It was said that even fish loved Francis. Whenever a fish was caught and he was nearby, he would return the fish to the water, warning it not to be caught again. It was reported that on several occasions the fish would linger awhile near the boat, listening to Francis preach, until he gave them permission to leave.

Francis and the Wolf of Gubbio

Perhaps the most famous story of Francis is when he tamed the wolf that was terrorizing the people of Gubbio. While Francis was staying in that town he learned of a wolf so ravenous that it was not only killing and eating animals, but people, too. The people took up arms and went after it, but those who encountered the wolf perished. Villagers became afraid to leave the city walls.

Francis had pity on the people and decided to go out and meet the wolf. He was desperately warned by the people, but he insisted that God would take care of him. A brave friar and several peasants accompanied Francis outside the city gate. But soon the peasants lost heart and said they would go no farther.

Francis and his companion began to walk on. Suddenly the wolf, jaws agape with saliva dripping, charged out of the woods at the couple. Undaunted and with fearless love, Francis made the Sign of the Cross towards it. The wolf slowed down, standing still and closed its mouth.

Then Francis called out to the creature: "Come to me, Brother Wolf. In the name of Christ, I order you not to hurt anyone." At that moment the wolf lowered its head and lay down at the saint's feet, meek as a lamb.

Francis explained to the wolf that he had been terrorizing the people, killing not only animals, but humans who are made in the image of God. "Brother Wolf," said Francis, "I want to make peace between you and the people of Gubbio. They will harm you no more and you must no longer harm them. All past crimes are to be forgiven."

The wolf showed its assent by moving its body and nodding its head. The saint then asked the wolf to make a pledge. As Francis extended his hand to receive the pledge, so the wolf extended its front paw and placed it into the saint's hand. Then Francis commanded the wolf to follow him into town to make a peace pact with the townspeople. The wolf meekly followed.

By the time they got to the town square, everyone was there to witness the miracle. With the wolf at his side, Francis gave the town a sermon on the wondrous and fearful love of God, calling them to repent from all their sins. Then he offered the townspeople peace, on behalf of the wolf. The townspeople promised in a loud voice to feed the wolf. Then Francis asked the wolf if it would live in peace under those terms. It bowed its head and twisted its body in a way that convinced everyone that it had accepted the pact. Then once again the wolf placed its paw in Francis' hand as a sign of the pact.

From that day on the people kept the pact they had made. The wolf lived for two years among the townspeople, going from door to door for food. It hurt no one and no one hurt it. Even the dogs did not bark at it. When the wolf finally died of old age, the people of Gubbio were sad. The wolf's peaceful ways had been a living reminder to them of the holiness of Francis and reality of Divine providence.

The teachings of Francis are best conveyed by the following simple prayer which he lived so well:

Rudra Shivananda

Lord, make me an instrument of Thy peace:
Where there is hatred, let me sow love;
Where there is injury, pardon;
Where there is discord, union;
Where there is doubt, faith;
Where there is despair, hope;
Where there is darkness, light!
Where there is sadness, joy.

O Divine Master, grant that I may not so much seek
To be consoled, as to console;
To be understood, as to understand;
To be loved, as to love;
For it is in giving that we receive,
It is in pardoning that we are pardoned,
And it is in dying that we are born to Eternal Life.

Nanak

Nanak was born on April 15, 1469 near Lahore in the Punjab, during a very turbulent and violent time in northern India, caused by the repeated invasions and occupations of Muslim kings. His father was in the warrior caste; but under the Muslims they were not allowed to be in the military, and so instead was a shopkeeper and record-keeper for a landlord, who had converted to Islam. Nanak learned arithmetic and accounting from his father, reading and writing in Hindi from a priest, and Persian and Arabic as well.

Even as a child, Nanak was precocious and cared not for material things, but had a tendency to give away his father's goods to the poor and often quarreled with him.

When Nanak was sixteen, his older sister's husband got him a job in the store of the regional governor. Two years later Nanak married the daughter of a Punjab merchant, and they had two sons. He would look after the store in the daytime and meditate long into the nights. All his free time was spent with ascetics and sages. All his spare money was given to take care of the ascetics, who had nothing.

On the November full moon of 1496, Nanak had a transformational experience. As was his custom, the first thing every morning, Nanak would bathe in a stream. However, on this day, after he had plunged into the water, he failed to re-appear, and his servant could find no trace of him. Fearing that his master had drowned, the servant enlisted the help of the townspeople to find him, but to no avail. After everyone had given up hope of ever seeing the young man again, on the third day after his mysterious disappearance, Nanak reappeared in the town, as if nothing had happened!

Nanak had been transformed and he started to teach. His message was simple:

- There is no Hindu; there is no Muslim which has several layers of meaning, implying human and religious unity and also that those who call themselves one or the other are not truly so. When the local Muslim religious leader complained about his message, Nanak sang that his devotees are ever joyous, for they learn how to end sorrow and sin.
- One must labor to earn and share one's earnings with others.

In 1499, together with a minstrel Mardana who had become his closest disciple, he left his post and began traveling. Everywhere he went he was seeing the aggressive spread of the Mohammedan faith. Nanak often joined the Muslims in their prayers. However, he suggested that their first prayer should be to speak the truth, the second to ask for lawfully earned daily bread, the third to practice charity, the fourth to purify the mind, and the fifth to adore and worship God.

Nanak preached against caste distinctions. He personally dined with those of low caste, and he raised the status of women.

He tried to moderate the excessive brutality of the Muslims against the Hindus by emphasized *gan* - singing praises of God, *dan* - charity for all, *ashnan* - purification by bathing, *seva* - serving humanity, and *simran* - constantly praying to God. Nanak himself often abstained from eating animal food.

After spending two years in the southwest Punjab, from 1501 to 1514 Nanak traveled to the southeast in India. In Delhi he and Mardana were arrested for violating an order against preaching in public; but their singing in jail caused such a disturbance that they were soon released. From 1515 to 1517 he was in the Himalayas and went as far as Tibet. About 1520 Nanak traveled to Mecca, probably by sea, and many believe he visited Baghdad on his way home that took him through Iran and Afghanistan.

While arriving outside Mecca, Nanak was tired and laid down for a rest. Muslim pilgrims were scandalized because they saw that he had his feet pointed toward the holy city, and were going to punish him. Gently, Nanak told them that he would move his feet, if they could show him in which direction God was not. They fell silent and treated him as a holy man.

The hymns of Nanak indicate that he witnessed the Muslim Babur's third invasion of the Punjab in the winter of 1521, for he complained about the raping of women and how Death had come disguised as the Mughal Babur. In the fourth invasion of 1524 Nanak saw the city of Lahore given over to death and violence for four hours. After the fifth invasion of 1526 Nanak lamented the dark age of the sword in which kings are butchers, and goodness has fled. He also referred to kings as tigers and their officials as dogs that eat carrion. The subjects blindly pay homage out of ignorance as if they were dead.

A wealthy devotee donated land on the bank of the Ravi, and the village of Kartarpur was built for Nanak and his disciples. Nanak lived there from 1522 until his death on September 22, 1539. Nanak did not consider himself an avatar or a prophet but a guru who could help people find God.

Amongst his devotees were two friends who lived in the same town. On the way to see their Guru, one of them came across a courtesan and fell under her charms, and from then on, while the sincere devotee went everyday to pay his respects to Nanak, the other one would visit the women instead. Soon after, the sincere devotee was pricked by a thorn, while the undisciplined one found a coin on the street on the way to the prostitute. This troubled the former, who asked his Guru for an explanation. Nanak smiled and responded: "Your friend was destined to come across a treasure, but because of his evil ways, the treasure was reduced to a single gold coin. On account of your past *karma*, you were going to be impaled with a stake, but because you disciplined and reformed yourself, this was reduced to a thorn's prick."

Nanak's songs were later collected together in the *Adi Granth* that became the scripture for the Sikh religion. His basic teaching about God is summarized in the *Mul Mantra*:

> *God is one,*
> *Truth is the Divine Name*
> *Creator,*
> *Fearless,*
> *Without ill-will,*
> *Immortal,*
> *Unborn,*
> *Self-existent,*
> *Realized by Divine grace*
> *through the Self-Realized Master.*

The *Mul Mantra* is followed by the longer *Jap Ji*, which Nanak wrote about 1520. *Jap Ji* means "great meditation for a new life." It begins by noting that God can not be comprehended by reason nor by outward silence, and one cannot buy contentment with all the riches in the world. The way to know the truth is to make God's will one's own. All things are manifestations of God's will, which is beyond description. By communing with the divine Word and meditating on God's glory one may find salvation by divine grace. The Word washes away all sin and sorrow and bestows virtue. By practicing the Word one rises into universal consciousness, develops understanding of the whole creation, transcends death, and also guides others. Yet no one can describe the condition of the one who has made God's will one's own. People carry their deeds with them wherever they go, because one reaps what one has sown. The highest religion is universal brotherhood that considers all equals.

Because all are equal, one should not fear any human being but only God. Nanak fostered community kitchens in his communities so that all devotees regardless of caste could eat free meals together. Attendance was also equally available to women.

Nanak sang that one should conquer one's mind, for overcoming self is victory over the world. Wealth and supernatural powers distract one from God. *Jap Ji* concludes:

> *Make continence your furnace, patience your smithy,*
> *The Master's word your anvil,*
> *and true knowledge your hammer.*
> *Make awe of God your bellows*
> *and with it kindle the fire of austerity,*
> *And in the crucible of love, melt the nectar Divine,*

The world operates by the two opposite principles of union and separation. Everyone is judged according to one's actions, through the divine law of *Karma*:

> *Air is the Master, Water the father,*
> *and the Earth the mother,*
> *Day and night are the two nursemaids*
> *in whose lap the whole world is at play.*
> *Our actions: good and evil,*
> *will be brought before Divine Law.*
> *By our own deeds, shall we move*
> *Closer to or further away from the Divine .*
> *Those who have communed with the Word,*
> *their toils shall end.*
> *And their faces shall flame with glory,*
> *Not only shall they have salvation,*
> *but many more shall find freedom through them.*

Nanak emphasized the oneness of God, the importance of repeating the divine Name and completely surrendering to God's will. He believed that only God and the Guru are without error. A record is kept of everyone's actions. The virtuous are treated well and remain in heaven, but the sinners transmigrate for the punishment that may educate them. Nanak advised his followers to give charity secretly and be humble. God frees people through the true Guru. Faithful disciples worship God patiently, shun evil, eat and drink moderately, and are detached from the world. Love and humility are the most essential qualities of worship. God's justice is impartial to all, rich or poor, high or low.

Nanak showed that the way by which all people could escape from the misery of a selfish life and reincarnation is by *ishvar pranidhan* or total surrender to the Divine. The divine order (*hukam* or *dharma*) can be perceived when the Guru awakens in the person the voice of God within. The sound of this Word (*shabada*) or Name (*nam*) of God can be heard in loving meditation so that the essence of God and the creation is communicated through human experience. By practicing this discipline (*simran*) the devotee ascends to higher levels until the ineffable oneness of God is attained.

Nanak rejected all external forms of rituals, ceremonies, caste distinctions, scriptures, and all the dualities of the human mind. He said of the sacred thread, the mark of a religious Hindu:

> *Let mercy be the cotton,*
> *Contentment the thread,*
> *Continence the knot,*
> *and Truth the twist.*
> *If you have a sacred thread like this,*
> *Do give it to me.*
> *It won't wear out or get soiled,*
> *Neither burn nor get lost.*
> *Blessed is the one who wears such a thread.*

To the Mohammedan, Nanak counseled:

> *Let compassion be your mosque,*
> *Devotion your prayer mat,*
> *Truth and fair play the Holy Qur'an,*
> *Let modesty be your circumcision*
> *And courtesy the fast of a muslim.*
> *Your conduct be the Kaaba,*
> *Rectitude your guide,*
> *And good deeds your creed and prayer.*

The inward way is open to all, including those with a family life. For Nanak the one God is both *nirguna* and *saguna*, meaning both absolute and conditioned, both manifest and unmanifest. The selfishness of lust, anger, avarice, attachment, and pride must be overcome. The Guru is the ladder or the vehicle by which one reaches God. Nanak recognized the law of *Karma* by which individuals reap what they sow, and the goal is to attain liberation from the cycle of reincarnation. The grace of God enables one to transcend the law of *Karma* and become free. Loving meditation on God is the way to do this. Like Jesus, Nanak compared the Name of God to a seed that must be planted in the field of the body, plowed by the mind through actions, irrigated with effort, leveled with contentment, and fenced with humility.

Nanak taught a disciplined ascent through five stages, called *simran*. The first is realizing one's connection with God and beginning discipline; the second is acquiring knowledge and understanding; the third is effort; the fourth is God's grace that comes to the fully devoted disciple; and the fifth is truth and the merging of the disciple into the one God. The discipline of *simran* means being devoted to the good and also implies good actions.

Mahatma Gandhi

Mohandas Karamchand Gandhi was born on October 2, 1869 in western India. His father was a local politician. At the age of 13 Mohandas was married to a girl his own age and after finishing his preliminary education, it was decided that he should go to England to study law. He joined the Inner Temple law college in London. In searching for a vegetarian restaurant he discovered its philosophy in Henry Salt's A Plea for Vegetarianism and became convinced. He organized a vegetarian club and met people with theosophical and altruistic interests. His first reading of the *Bhagavad-Gita* was in Edwin Arnold's poetic translation The Song Celestial. This classic of the *sanatana dharma* and the Sermon on the Mount later became his bibles and spiritual guidebooks. He memorized the *Gita* during his daily tooth-brushing and often recited its original Sanskrit at his prayer meetings.

When Gandhi returned to India in 1891 he was not successful at breaking into the legal profession due to his innate shyness. Instead he took an opportunity to represent an Indian firm South Africa for a year. As a lawyer Gandhi did his best to discover the facts and get the parties to accept arbitration and compromise in order to settle out of court. After solving a difficult case in this way he was elated and commented, "I had learnt to find out the better side of human nature and to enter men's hearts. I realized that the true function of a lawyer was to unite parties riven asunder." He also insisted on receiving the truth from his clients, and if he found out that they had lied he would drop their cases. He believed that the lawyer's duty was to help the court discover the truth, not to try to prove the guilty innocent.

South Africa was then rampant in racial discrimination of a high order and his experiences there awakened his social conscience. When he was ordered to remove his turban in court, he refused. He was thrown out of a first-class railway compartment; On another occasion, he was beaten for refusing to move to the footboard of a stage-coach for the sake of a European passenger.

At the end of the year during a farewell party before he was to sail for India, Gandhi noticed in the newspaper that a bill was being proposed that would deprive Indians of the vote. His friends urged him to stay and lead the fight for their rights in South Africa. Gandhi founded the Natal Indian Congress in 1894, and their efforts were given considerable notice by the press. When he returned from fetching his family from India in January 1897 the South Africans tried to stop him from landing by bribing and threatening the ship-owner. The waiting mob recognized Gandhi, and some whites began to hit his face and body until the Police Superintendent's wife came to his rescue. The mob threatened to lynch him, but Gandhi escaped in a disguise. Later he refused to prosecute anyone, holding to the principle of self-restraint in regard to a personal wrong. Gandhi ended up spending twenty years in South Africa.

After his early marriage, he had been sexually active, but in his thirties, he experimented with celibacy and in 1906 took the *brahmacharya* vow and became a celibate for the rest of his life. The first use of civil disobedience on a mass scale came in September 1906. The Transvaal government wanted to register the entire Indian population. The Indians held a mass meeting in the Imperial Theatre of Johannesburg; they were angry at the humiliating ordinance, and some threatened a violent response if put to the test. However, they decided as a group to refuse to comply with the registration provisions. Yet Gandhi suggested that they take a pledge in the name of God; even though they were Hindus and Moslems they all believed in one and the same God. Every one of the nearly three thousand Indians present took the solemn pledge.

Gandhi decided to call this technique of refusing to submit to injustice *Satyagraha* which means literally "holding to the truth."

Gandhi declared to his followers that a *Satyagrahi* (one who follows the principles of *Satyagraha*) must be fearless and always trust his opponent, "for an implicit trust in human nature is the very essence of his creed." *Satyagraha* uncovers hidden motives and reveals the truth - even if it results in the opponent's falseness, this will be more sharply felt and will be more clearly seen, and the opponent must continually be given the opportunity to be true. While reading in jail Gandhi discovered Thoreau's Civil Disobedience and the works of Tolstoy. He was impressed and "began to realize more and more the infinite possibilities of universal love."

One week after the pledge Asiatic women were excused from having to register. When the Transvaal government finally put the Asiatic Registration Act into effect in 1907, Gandhi and several other Indians were arrested. He was given only two months without hard labor, and he spent the time reading. Yet during his life Gandhi would spend a total of more than six and a half years in jail. Gandhi was called to meet with the South African leader, General Jan Christiaan Smuts, and they agreed on a compromise.

As the protest movement for Indian rights in South Africa grew - at one point out of the 13,000 Indians in the province 2,500 Indians were in jail, while 6,000 had fled. In being civil to the opponents during the disobedience Gandhi developed the use of *ahimsa*, which means "nonviolence." Since we are all one spiritually, to hurt or attack another person is to attack oneself. **Though we may attack an unjust system, we must always love the persons involved. Thus "*ahimsa* is the basis of the search for truth."**

In 1913, three issues brought the quest for Indian rights in South Africa to another crisis - the tax on ex-serfs, the ban on Asiatic immigrants, and the invalidating of all but Christian marriages. In November Gandhi led a march of over two thousand people, and was arrested and released on bail, arrested again and released, and arrested once more all within four days. He was sentenced to three months' hard labor, but the strikes and demonstrations went on with about 50,000 indentured laborers on strike and thousands of free Indians in prison. The Christian missionary Charles F. Andrews donated all his money to the movement. Gandhi and the other leaders were released and announced another march. However, Gandhi refused to take advantage of a railway strike by white employees and called off the march in spite of Smut's broken pledge in 1908. "Forgiveness is the ornament of the brave," Gandhi explained. Finally by negotiation the issues were resolved: all marriages regardless of religion were valid; the tax on indentured laborers was canceled including arrears; Indians were allowed to move more freely. Gandhi began to feel that the power of the *Satyagraha* method could transform modern civilization. "It is a force which, if it became universal, would revolutionize social ideals and do away with despotisms and the ever-growing militarism under which the nations of the West are groaning and are being almost crushed to death, and which fairly promises to overwhelm even the nations of the East." Smuts expressed his respect for Gandhi and his gentle but powerful methods which had made him realize that the law had to be repealed.

Meanwhile India was still suffering under British colonial rule. In 1909 Gandhi had written *Hind Swaraj* which means 'Indian Self-Rule.' In this essay against the corruption of Western civilization Gandhi suggested that India could gain its independence by nonviolent means and self-reliance. He rejected violence and declared that soul force or love is what keeps people together in peace and harmony. History ignores the peaceful qualities but takes note of the interruptions and violations which disrupt civilization. Gandhi returned to India in 1915 and again supported the British during the First World War by raising and leading an ambulance corps.

The great poet and Nobel laureate Rabindranath Tagore gave Gandhi the title *Mahatma* meaning 'Great Soul.' Gandhi founded the *Satyagraha* Ashram for his family and co-workers near the textile city of Ahmedabad. When a family of untouchables asked to live in the ashram, Gandhi admitted them. Orthodox Hindus believed this polluted them, and refused to help. Funds ran out, and Gandhi was ready to live in the untouchable slums if necessary, but an anonymous benefactor donated enough money to last a year. To help change people's attitudes about these unfortunate pariahs, Gandhi renamed them *Harijans* or 'Children of God.'

India had cooperated with Britain during the first World War, and instead of gaining greater freedom as promised, civil liberties were being curtailed. In 1919 Gandhi decided to call for a one-day general strike on all economic activity. Many signed the *Satyagraha* pledge, and Gandhi suggested making "a continuous and persistent effort to return good for evil." However this philosophy was not well understood by the masses, and violence erupted in various places, prompting him to call off the campaign. In one infamous incident General Dyer had ordered his soldiers to fire into a crowd of women and children resting in cul-de-sac, wounding 1,137 and killing 379. The investigative report indicated that he was less concerned with dispersing the crowd and more intent on "producing a sufficient moral effect from a military point of view." The report concluded that the moral effect was quite opposite from the one intended.

In 1920 Gandhi initiated a nation-wide campaign of non-cooperation with the British government, which for the peasant meant non-payment of taxes and no buying of liquor since the government gained revenue from its sale. Gandhi traveled throughout India addressing mass meetings. He urged people to spin their own cloth and designed a Congress flag with a spinning wheel in the center. By January 1922 thirty thousand Indians had been jailed for civil disobedience. Some nationalist patriots urged revolution, but Gandhi would never forsake nonviolence. In March the British Viceroy ordered Gandhi's arrest. This was the only time that the British allowed him a trial. He made no apology and explained, "In my opinion, non-cooperation with evil is as much a duty as is cooperation with good." The judge sentenced him to six years and hoped the government would reduce the term. He was in fact released after twenty-two months when he had an appendectomy.

Perhaps the greatest block to Indian unity and self government was the conflict between Hindus and Moslems. In 1924 Gandhi went on a twenty-one day fast to bridge this strife. He pleaded for unity in diversity, religious tolerance, and love for one another.

During the late 1920s Gandhi wrote an autobiography which he called his experiments with truth. It is quite candid and humble in the way he examines his faults and his efforts to overcome them.

In his speeches he pointed out his five-point program on the fingers of his hand: equality for untouchables, spinning, no alcohol or drugs, Hindu-Moslem friendship, and equality for women. They were all connected to the wrist which stood for nonviolence. Finally in 1928 he announced a *Satyagraha* campaign in Bardoli against a 22% increase in British imposed taxes. Refusing to pay taxes the people had their possessions confiscated and some were driven off their land, but they remained nonviolent. It lasted several months, and hundreds were arrested. Finally the government gave in and agreed to cancel the tax increase, release all prisoners, and return confiscated land and property; the peasants agreed to pay their taxes at the previous rate.

The Indian Congress wanted self-government and considered war for independence. Gandhi naturally refused to support a war but declared that if India was not free under Dominion Status by the end of 1929, then he would demand independence. Consequently in 1930 he informed the Viceroy that civil disobedience would begin on March 11. "My ambition is no less than to convert the British people through nonviolence, and thus make them see the wrong they have done to India. I do not seek to harm your people."

Gandhi decided to disobey the Salt Laws which forbade Indians from making their own salt - this barbarous British monopoly especially struck at the poor. Beginning with seventy-eight members of his ashram Gandhi led a two-hundred mile march to the sea over twenty-four days. Thousands had gathered at the start, and several thousands joined them on the march. First Gandhi and then others all along the seacoast gathered some salt water in pans to dry it. In Bombay the Congress had salt pans on their roof – sixty-thousand people assembled, and hundreds were arrested. At Karachi where fifty thousand watched the salt being made, the crowd was so thick that the police could make no arrests. The jails were filled with at least sixty thousand offenders. Amazingly enough there was practically no violence at all - the people did not want Gandhi to cancel the movement. Gandhi was arrested.

According to an eye-witness account by the reporter Webb Miller, about two thousand five hundred volunteers continued to march into a salt factory until beaten down with steel-shod rods by the four hundred police, but they did not try to fight back. Such incidents made Tagore declare that Europe had lost her moral prestige in Asia. Soon more than one hundred thousand Indians were in prison, including almost all the leaders.

Gandhi was called to a meeting with Viceroy Irwin in 1931, and they came to an agreement in March. Civil disobedience was called off; prisoners were released; salt manufacture was permitted on the coast; Congress leaders would attend the next Round Table Conference in London.

Progress was slow – the British kept stalling and Gandhi continued to preach a nonviolent revolution for India. In 1942 he and other leaders were arrested. He decided to fast again - he barely survived.

When the war ended he asserted the need for "a real peace based on the freedom and equality of all races and nations." He said, "Violence is bred by inequality, nonviolence by equality."

Independence for India was now imminent, but Jinnah the Moslem leader was holding out for the creation of a separate state of Pakistan. Gandhi prayed for unity and tolerance, and he even read from the Koran at his prayer meetings. Hindus attacked him because they thought he was partial to Moslems, and Moslems demanded he let them have Pakistan. Gandhi went to Calcutta to calm the Hindu-Moslem strife and violence. Once more he fasted until the community leaders signed a pledge to keep the peace - before they signed he warned them that if they broke their word he would fast until he died. His last fast in January 1948 also did much to heal the conflicts between the Hindus and the Moslems over the division into two countries which left minorities in both nations. Although this religious hatred saddened Gandhi, India had gained her independence on August 15, 1947 accomplishing the greatest nonviolent revolution in the history of the world.

This great exponent of love and nonviolence was assassinated by an outraged Hindu on January 30, 1948 at a prayer meeting. With his last breath the Mahatma chanted the name of God.

Albert Einstein declared that Gandhi showed how someone could win allegiance, "not merely by the cunning game of political fraud and trickery, but through the living example of a morally exalted way of life." Einstein considered Gandhi to be the most enlightened statesman of their time, and he predicted, "The problem of bringing peace to the world on a supranational basis will be solved only by employing Gandhi's method on a large scale." The Encyclopedia Britannica summarizes Gandhi's significance with the statement, "He was the catalyst if not the initiator of three of the major revolutions of the 20th century: the revolutions against colonialism, racism, and violence."

His Teaching: The marriage of Truth and Nonviolence

Satyagraha means literally holding on to the Truth, with the understanding that *Sat* is more than conceptual truth but means also being, existence, reality - ultimately we must realize that our spiritual being-ness as the essence of Truth as a reality greater than any concept of the mind. Thus the term "soul-force" conveys the idea of employing our spiritual energies. For the Mahatma this Truth or spiritual reality is the goal, and the means to the goal must be as pure and loving as possible. *Ahimsa* therefore is the way of acting without hurting anyone or inflicting oneself against another spiritual being. We may hate an injustice for the harm that it brings to people, but we must always love all the people involved out of respect for human dignity. *Satyagraha* attempts to awaken an awareness of the truth about the injustice in the perpetrators, and by *ahimsa* this is done without hurting them. Since humans are fallible and we cannot be sure we are judging accurately, it behooves us to refrain from punishing. *Ahimsa* is then an essential safeguard in the quest for truth and justice.

To counter a popular misunderstanding, Gandhi explained that Satyagraha was not a method for the weak, like passive resistance, but "a weapon of the strong and excludes the use of violence in any shape or form." *Satyagraha* demands the truth and can be applied in relation to one's family, rulers, fellow citizens, or even the whole world. Gandhi elucidates three necessary conditions for its success application:

- The *Satyagrahi* should not have any hatred in his heart against the opponent.
- The issue must be true and substantial.
- The *Satyagrahi* must be prepared to suffer until the end for his cause.

The Mahatma emphasized the austerity or *tapas* of self-suffering rather than inflicting suffering on others. By undergoing suffering to reveal the injustice the *Satya*grahi strives to reach the consciences of people. *Satyagraha* does not try to coerce anyone but rather to convert by persuasion, to reach the reason through the heart.

> *If man will only realize*
> *that it is unmanly to obey laws that are unjust,*
> *no man's tyranny will enslave him.*

Satyagraha requires self-discipline, self control, and self-purification, and *Satyagrahis* must always make the distinction between the evil and the evil-doer. They must overcome evil with good, hatred with love, anger with patience, untruth with truth, and violence with *ahimsa*. This takes a perfect person for complete success, and therefore training and education are essential to even make it workable. Gandhi emphasizes that every child "should know what the soul is, what truth is, what love is, what powers are latent in the soul."

> *Nonviolence is the law of our species*
> *as violence is the law of the brute.*
> *The spirit lies dormant in the brute,*
> *and he knows no law but that of physical might.*
> *The dignity of man requires obedience to a higher law -*
> *to the strength of the spirit.*

From his experience Gandhi believed that those who wished to serve their country through Satyagraha should "observe perfect chastity, adopt poverty, follow truth, and cultivate fearlessness." It is through fearlessness that we can have the courage to renounce all harmful weapons, filling and surrounding ourselves with the spiritual protection of a loving and peaceful consciousness.

> *For self-defense, I would restore the spiritual culture.*
> *The best and most lasting self-defense is self-purification.*

Non-cooperation is a comprehensive policy used by people when they can no longer in good conscience participate in or support a government that has become oppressive, unjust, and violent. Although *Satyagrahis* do not attack the wrong-doer, it is their responsibility not to promote or support the wrong actions. Thus non-cooperators withdraw from government positions, renounce government programs and services, and refuse to pay taxes to the offending government. While challenging the power of the state in this way non-cooperators have the opportunity to learn greater self-reliance. Gandhi held that non-cooperation with an unjust government was not only an inherent right but as much a duty as is cooperation with a just government.

Ahimsa or nonviolence is absolutely essential to Gandhi's civil disobedience. *Satyagrahis* were expected to give their lives in efforts to quell violence if it erupted. Gandhi interpreted *ahimsa* broadly as refraining from anything at all harmful:

> *The principle of ahimsa is hurt by every evil thought, by undue haste, by lying, by hatred, by wishing ill to anybody. It is also violated by our holding on to what the world needs.*

This means that even greed and avarice can violate *ahimsa*. Nonviolence has a great spiritual power, but the slightest use of violence can taint a just cause. The strength is not physical but comes from spiritual will, which can only be harnessed through self-knowledge:

> *There can be no inward peace without true knowledge*

The Mahatma himself summarized the implications of nonviolence as follows:

- Nonviolence is the law of the human race and is infinitely greater than and superior to brute force.
- In the last resort it does not avail to those who do not possess a living faith in the God of Love.
- Nonviolence affords the fullest protection to one's self-respect and sense of honor, but not always to possession of land or movable property, though its habitual practice does prove a better bulwark than the possession of armed men to defend them. Nonviolence, in the very nature of things, is of no assistance in the defense of ill-gotten gains and immoral acts.
- Individuals or nations who would practice nonviolence must be prepared to sacrifice (nations to the last man) their all except for honor. It is, therefore, inconsistent with the possession of other people's countries, i.e., modern imperialism, which is frankly based on force for its defense.
- Nonviolence is a power which can be wielded equally by all-children, young men and women or grown-up people, provided they have a living faith in the God of Love and have therefore equal love for all mankind. When nonviolence is accepted as the law of life it must pervade the whole being and not be applied to isolated acts.
- It is a profound error to suppose that whilst the law is good enough for individuals it is not for masses of mankind.

Mahatma Gandhi has shown that the great spiritual truths of mankind can be successfully applied to all our activities, even in the active righting of wrongs, without violating the moral precepts.

Martin Luther King

With nonviolent resistance,
no individual or group need submit to any wrong,
nor need anyone resort to violence in order to right a wrong.

Martin Luther King Jr. was born on January 15, 1929 in Atlanta, Georgia and was named after his father who was a successful Baptist preacher. From 1956 until his death in 1968, he was the foremost leader in black Americans' non-violent quest for civil rights and a better life. King started at Morehouse College in Atlanta when he was only 15, and he graduated four years later. Choosing the ministry over medicine and law, he attended Crozer Theological Seminary in Pennsylvania for three years. While there he heard Mordecai Johnson lecture on Gandhi. He was so moved by the idea of refusing to cooperate with an evil system that he went out and bought every book he could find on Gandhi and nonviolence.

After studying Gandhi, King realized that the love ethic of Jesus could go beyond individuals and be applied to the conflicts of racial groups and nations. He discovered the method for social reform in Gandhi's love force (*Satyagraha*) and nonviolence. After being elected student body president and graduating first in his class at Crozer, King moved on to Boston University where he earned his Ph.D. in Theology. In 1953 he married Coretta Scott, a student of music, and they eventually had four children. Believing in the guidance of a personal God and equipped with the techniques of nonviolence, King accepted a pastorate in Montgomery, Alabama, planning to help his people achieve social justice.

On May 17, 1954 the United States Supreme Court had declared, "Separate educational facilities are inherently unequal," and in 1955 the same Court ordered all public schools to be desegregated "with all deliberate speed." A fifteen-year-old girl had been arrested for refusing to give up her seat to a white passenger on the bus, and then on December 1955 Mrs. Rosa Parks felt her feet were too tired for her to stand up for a white man who had boarded after her. The bus driver ordered her to stand up and give her seat to the white man, but she refused. She was arrested and taken to the courthouse. Over forty black leaders showed up at King's church, and they agreed to boycott the buses on the following Monday. Leaflets were copied and distributed announcing these actions. Committees were organized, and alternative transportation was arranged. King thought of the movement as a massive non-cooperation against an evil system. The word spread, and on Monday morning the Montgomery buses were practically empty except for a few white passengers.

King spoke for the hearts of many when he declared that they were "tired of being segregated and humiliated," and affirmed that their only alternative was to protest for freedom and justice. Christian love and non-violent principles provided the basis for his advice. He said, "No one must be intimidated to keep them from riding the buses. Our method must be persuasion, not coercion. We will only say to the people: Let your conscience be your guide." He concluded his speech, "If you will protest courageously, and yet with dignity and Christian love, future historians will say, that there lived a great people - a black people - who injected new meaning and dignity into the veins of civilization. This is our challenge and our overwhelming responsibility." During the mass meeting, the following demands were unanimously approved at the mass meeting:

- courteous treatment by bus operators
- passengers to be seated on a first-come, first-served basis with Negroes in the back and whites in the front
- Negro bus drivers to be employed in predominantly Negro routes.

In his book Stride Toward Freedom, King explained how Christian love and non-violent methods guided the movement. In weekly meetings he would emphasize that the use of violence would be both impractical and immoral:

> *Hate begets hate; violence begets violence;*
> *toughness begets a greater toughness.*
> *We must meet the forces of hate with the power of love;*
> *we must meet physical force with soul force.*
> *Our aim must never be to defeat or*
> *humiliate the white man,*
> *but to win his friendship and understanding.*

To King nonviolence was a way of life, but he was glad that the black people were willing to accept it as a method; he presented it simply as Christianity in action.

Again, in Stride Toward Freedom King elucidates six key points about the philosophy of nonviolence.

- It is not based on cowardice; although it may seem passive physically, it is spiritually active, requiring the courage to stand up against injustice.
- Nonviolence does not seek to defeat the opponent but rather to win his understanding to create "the beloved community."
- The attack is directed at the evil not at the people who are doing the evil; for King the conflict was not between whites and blacks but between justice and injustice.
- In nonviolence there is a willingness to accept suffering without retaliating.
- Not only is physical violence avoided but also spiritual violence; love replaces hatred.
- Nonviolence has faith that justice will prevail.

King was persecuted for years – he was arrested in January for driving 30 in a 25 mile-per-hour zone, even though he was driving very carefully since he was aware of being followed. The Kings' house was bombed; however, Coretta and a friend had escaped injury by moving quickly to the back of the house. Martin rushed home from his meeting, and a furious mob gathered outside. He calmed them down and advised them to put down their weapons and go home. He said, "We cannot solve this problem through retaliatory violence. We must meet violence with nonviolence.... We must meet hate with love." King quieted the crowd. His presence and words had prevented a bloody riot. Even though he often received threatening phone calls, true to his beliefs, King would not allow a weapon in his house.

On June 4, 1956 a federal court held that bus segregation was unconstitutional. However, the city attorneys appealed to the Supreme Court. The Montgomery attorney arrested King and other black leaders for violating an old law against boycotts. While they were in a Montgomery court on this charge, the Supreme Court affirmed the decision declaring Alabama's state and local laws requiring segregation on buses unconstitutional.

Meetings were held to prepare the people for integration of the buses. Training sessions in non-violent techniques enabled "actors" to play out different roles before a critical audience which would discuss the results. Integrated bus suggestions were printed which recommended "complete nonviolence in word and action" and the admonition, "Be loving enough to absorb evil and understanding enough to turn an enemy into a friend." A few days before Christmas, after more than a year's boycott, the black ministers of Montgomery led the way in riding integrated buses.

When the Eisenhower Administration failed to respond to a call for dialog, King organized a 'Prayer Pilgrimage of Freedom' which drew thirty-seven thousand marchers to the Lincoln Memorial in

Washington on May 17,1957. King led the cry of blacks for the ballot so that they could participate more fully in the legislative process.

Echoing the philosophy of Gandhi, in 1958 Stride Toward Freedom came out calling for a militant and non-violent mass movement. King suggests in this book that if they remain non-violent, then public opinion will be magnetically attracted to them rather than to the instigators of violence. A non-violent mass movement is power under discipline seeking justice. He summarizes his nonviolent intentions this way:

> *We will take direct action against injustice*
> *without waiting for other agencies to act.*
> *We will not obey unjust laws*
> *or submit to unjust practices.*
> *We will do this peacefully, openly, cheerfully*
> *because our aim is to persuade.*
> *We adopt the means of nonviolence*
> *because our end is a community at peace with itself.*
> *We will try to persuade with our words,*
> *but if our words fail,*
> *we will try to persuade with our acts.*
> *We will always be willing to talk*
> *and seek fair compromise,*
> *but we are ready to suffer, when necessary*
> *and even risk our lives*
> *to become witnesses to the truth as we see it.*

He points out that nonviolence first affects the hearts of those committed to it, gives them greater self-respect and courage, and then it stirs the conscience of the opponents until reconciliation is achieved. In a world of ballistic missiles he declares, "Today the choice is no longer between violence and nonviolence. It is either nonviolence or nonexistence."

While autographing copies of his book in New York, a woman stabbed King in the chest with a sharp letter opener. He remained calm and waited for a surgeon to remove the knife-like weapon. Its point had been touching his aorta, and he was told that if he had merely sneezed he might have died.

In February 1959 Martin Luther King made a pilgrimage to India and returned even more confirmed in the principles of nonviolence. On the first of December, King called for "a broad, bold advance of the southern campaign for equality." In 1960 student activists organized numerous sit-ins at lunch counters in order to end discrimination and the Student Nonviolent Coordinating Committee (SNCC) was formed. King and thirty-six others were arrested for sitting at the lunch counter in Rich's Department Store in Atlanta. The judge sentenced King to six months hard labor. This was on October 25, and the presidential election was only days away - John Kennedy and his brother Robert made some phone calls urging King's release.

In 1963, many volunteers came forward, for the Birmingham protests and the movement grew into a non-violent army. Each volunteer signed the following Commitment Card:

> I hereby pledge myself - my person and body - to the nonviolent movement. Therefore I will keep the following ten commandments:
>
> 1. Meditate daily on the teachings and life of Jesus.
> 2. Remember always that the nonviolent movement in Birmingham seeks justice and reconciliation - not victory.
> 3. Walk and talk in the manner of love, for God is love.
> 4. Pray daily to be used by God in order that all men might be free.
> 5. Sacrifice personal wishes in order that all men might be free.

6. Observe with both friend and foe the ordinary rules of courtesy.
7. Seek to perform regular service for others and for the world.
8. Refrain from the violence of fist, tongue, or heart.
9. Strive to be in good spiritual and bodily health.
10. Follow the directions of the movement and of the captain on a demonstration.

After being arrested again, he wrote on scraps of paper his famous letter from a Birmingham jail in which he responded to public charges that his actions were "unwise and untimely." He explained that he came to Birmingham because of the injustice there. They had gone through the four basic steps of a non-violent campaign: collection of facts about injustice, negotiation, self-purification, and direct action. He stated the truth, "We know through painful experience that freedom is never voluntarily given by the oppressor; it must be demanded by the oppressed." He quoted St. Augustine who said that "an unjust law is no law at all." Segregation is unjust because it damages the personality and creates false concepts of superiority and inferiority. To break an unjust law "openly, lovingly, and with a willingness to accept the penalty" is to express respect for real justice. He pointed out that what Hitler did in Germany was "legal," while aiding or comforting a Jew was "illegal." Nonviolence offers a creative outlet for repressed emotions which might otherwise result in violence.

After further thousands were jailed, an agreement was reached granting the major demands: desegregation of lunch counters, rest rooms, fitting rooms, and drinking fountains; upgrading and hiring of blacks on a non-discriminatory basis; release of all jailed persons; establishing communications between black and white leaders. Soon after, the Supreme Court decided that demonstrations against segregated institutions are legal. Justice had triumphed.

Two hundred fifty thousand people, about a third of them white, congregated at the Lincoln Memorial on August 28, 1963, to put pressure on the US Congress to pass President Kennedy's Civil Rights Bill. King was introduced as the "moral leader of the nation." The great crowd's response inspired him, and he put aside his text and began to speak of his dream of equality, brotherhood, and freedom - a dream where people are not judged by their skin color but by their character. He tolled the bell of freedom so that it would ring out all across the land.

On July 2, 1964 King personally witnessed President Lyndon Johnson's signing of the Civil Rights law. At the age thirty-five Martin Luther King became the youngest person ever to receive a Nobel Prize. He accepted the prestigious award for peace on behalf of the Movement, saying it was "a profound recognition that nonviolence is the answer to the crucial political and racial questions of our time-the need for man to overcome oppression without resorting to violence."

True to his conscience, and in spite of opposition from his fellow civil rights leaders, King spoke out against the Vietnam War. Many civil rights leaders considered his denunciation of Johnson's Vietnam policy a mistake. In January 1967, he declared, "The promises of the Great Society have been shot down on the battlefields of Vietnam.... We must combine the fervor of the Civil Rights Movement with the peace movement." He proposed a five-point peace program for Vietnam: beginning with an end to the bombing.

King believed that the root cause of both racial hatred and war was fear. He hoped that the greatest application of the non-violent methods used in the civil rights movement would be for world peace. "Do we have the morality and courage required to live together as brothers and not be afraid?" he asked. If we want mankind to survive, then we must find an alternative to war. Since modern weapons are calamitous, he suggested "that the philosophy and strategy of nonviolence become immediately a subject for study and for serious experimentation in every field of human conflict, by no means excluding the relations between nations." He had faith that we can end war and violence as long as we do not succumb to fear of the weapons we have created. Ultimately there must be a world-wide fellowship based on unconditional love for all people.

In 1968 Martin Luther King was preparing a massive Poor People's Campaign for whites as well as blacks when he was called to Memphis to assist with a strike of the sanitation workers. Two thousand people at Clayborn Temple wanted to hear him speak. He declared his support for their cause, but then he began to reflect about the threats made against his life. He confessed that he would like a long life, but his main concern was to do God's will. Like Moses, he was glad that he had been to the mountain top and seen the Promised Land.

The next day, April 4, 1968, Martin Luther King, Jr. was shot and killed. He had already requested a simple eulogy two months before when he had said, "I'd like someone to mention that day that Martin Luther King, Jr., tried to give his life serving others. I'd like somebody to say that day that Martin Luther King, Jr., tried to love somebody. I want you to be able to say that day that I did try to feed the hungry. I want you to be able to say that day that I did try in my life to clothe the naked. I want you to say on that day that I did try in my life to visit those who were in prison. And I want you to say that I tried to love and serve humanity."

The aftermath of nonviolence is reconciliation
and the creation of the beloved community.

Part 3
Tools for Transformation

Affirmations

An affirmation is a positive thought or statement that you repeat to yourself and implant in your inner consciousness as a source of inspiration for your present and future actions. Once secured in your subconscious mind, it guides your thoughts and actions in a chosen direction. You can use the power of affirmations to overcome certain undesirable traits and negative and habitual thought patterns in your mind or deal with some weakness in your personality affirmatively. They are powerful aids to the practice of *yama*.

There is a firm basis for the use of affirmations in the *yogic* process. The recipe for dealing with negative thoughts and obstructions that arise in the course of spiritual life has been succinctly given by the sage Patanjali in his Yoga Sutras II.33,34:

> *When the mind is disturbed by negative thoughts, the remedy is to constantly think of the opposite positive thoughts. As negative thoughts, emotions and actions, such as violence and so forth are done, caused to be done, or approved, whether arising from greed, anger or infatuation, whether present in mild, medium or intense degree, resulting in endless pain and ignorance; so there is a necessity or the yogi to cultivate the opposite.*

Using positive affirmations you can instruct your body and mind to act in a certain way. You can overcome the barriers that stand in between you and your true Self. You can send subtle thought forces into your consciousness and powerfully alter your thinking and behavior. Using positive affirmations, you can heal yourself in astonishing ways. You can stay motivated and focused on your path to spiritual enlightenment. You can truly transform your personality and make yourself more acceptable and at peace with yourself, overcoming many problems in your life, problems that exist because of some inherent deficiency or debility with your attitude, behavior or thinking, as a result of your *karmic* load.

Positive affirmations may not get you every thing you want in your life, but they can help you establish an environment in which you have greater opportunities to shape your life and alter the course of your actions. They can help you overcome the feelings of frustration and helplessness and make you feel confident, self reliant and responsible for your actions and thoughts. You can face the challenges of your life more confidently and with the conviction that you're not a mere pawn in the hands of some unknown fate. You can practically do anything that's humanly possible and within the field of your reality. It is possible to use affirmations for goals which are not particularly spiritually oriented, but such changes in life direction are generally band-aids which do not address the fundamental issues, which are generally *karmic* and spiritual, and therefore it is advisable to put more of your energy to solving these ultimate problems.

The characteristics of successful affirmations:

Following are some of the suggestions on how to make your affirmation work for you and bring success and happiness in your daily life:

- The affirmation should be appropriate to the problem that you want to deal with.

- Use words that focus on the end result desired.

- Repeat the affirmation regularly until it is firmly integrated with your consciousness and become part of your natural response to the intended problem.

- Associate your affirmation consciously and persistently with the problem you want to resolve.

- Balance your negative thought or fear with the positive affirmation

- Write the affirmation down on a paper or some book and keep it within easy reach.

- Memorize the affirmation for easy repetition.

- Start your day with positive affirmations and remember them before you go to bed. During the day, use them on as many occasions as you can, and definitely when you need them most - when there is a need to reinforce a desired behavior or state of mind or counter a problem or situation you are facing.

- Keep your affirmation simple, using action words that invoke positive imagery and appeal to your mind and sense directly.

- Make your affirmations personal and in first person. Feel the need for them strongly. Experience the sense of responsibility as you think of them.

- Use positive words only. Avoid negative expressions. Say, "I'm achieving this state of mind or reality," instead of "I don't want to be like this or that or I don't want to do this or that."

- Act as if your affirmations are already working and yielding positive results. Express your gratitude to the Divine.

- Add the power of visualization to the force of your affirmations. Visualize how your affirmations can change your life and your personality.

- Use the power of *Yoga Nidra* to create the environment for the most effective seeding of the affirmation on the receptive consciousness.

There are appropriate affirmations that help in the practice of the self-restraints of *yama*. It is difficult for most of us to practice *ahimsa* or nonviolence in thought, word or deed, since we are prone to anger and fear, which requires the antidote of love. The same situation exists for the other four restraints.

Yoga Nidra

This is a very powerful technique that goes beyond what is called a relaxation technique. It puts the *yogi* in touch with his consciousness from the lowest to the highest aspects.

This technique is used as:
- A healing and restorative "yogic sleep", in which awareness is maintained throughout.
- As an aid for the penetration and effectiveness of positive intent or affirmations.
- As an aid to mindfulness to attain to a state of awareness of the true Self
- As a means to eliminate the habit patterns caused by the activated or *Parabda Karma*.

> *Yogis use Yoga Nidra*
> *to eliminate samskaras,*
> *the fuel for karma.*

Samskaras are the deep seated habit patterns embedded in our causal body as a result of the *karma* which has been activated for the present life. All our thoughts, emotions, images, and sensations in the waking, sleeping and dreaming states are conditioned by our *samskaras* or predispositions.

Yoga Nidra is a tool for examining, attenuating, and eliminating those habit patterns or *samskaras*, which limit us from achieving freedom. Habitual negative actions, normally arising from these deep impressions can thus be reduced and eliminated through the appropriate practice.

In the Waking state, thought patterns can be troubling. In the Dream state, they can form trains of thoughts that seem to drag you around. However, imagine that you could observe your thought patterns when they were not active, when they were in a latent, sleeping form, while you were awake. Then they would not disturb or distract you. This is what happens in *Yoga Nidra*. The paradox is that while they are not in active form, they are still there. This can be difficult to conceptualize, but this is as close as we can get, to just say they are in a latent form.

As an analogy, imagine a photo on the screen of your computer. It might be a picture you find pleasing or offensive. However, imagine that you saw a print of the binary numbers, all of the zeros and ones, that represent the same picture in the memory of your hard disk. There would be no reaction whatsoever. They would just be a bunch of numbers, without any emotional charge to them. This is what happens when witnessing *samskaras* while you are in *Yoga Nidra*. There may be subtle traces of emotions, but they are very, very subtle, and do not seem to have the charge of active desires, wants, wishes, dislikes, or aversions.

By witnessing the *samskaras* in the state of *Yoga Nidra*, a certain **transformation** happens. They start to lose their coloring of attraction and aversion. They start to weaken, and are less and less able to later control our thoughts and actions. In this way, we use *Yoga Nidra* to reduce or soften the impact of our *samskaras* that play out in our daily lives like a series of disturbing software programs over which we have no control.

Through the continued practice and deepening of *Yoga Nidra*, there is an ever increasing awareness that, "I am not my thoughts!" In *Yoga Nidra*, you can experience a state of consciousness subsuming, or prior to all of the active mental process, both conscious and that which is normally unconscious – it is called the *turya* or the fourth state - the doorway to the awareness that still operates beyond all of the levels of mind, that leads to realization of the center of consciousness, or True Self.

It takes a lot of practice and the achievement of self-realization to reach the state of *turya* during *Yoga Nidra*. However, there are no barriers to achieving the states of deep relaxation in which the effective use of affirmations in the suggestive states that penetrate all levels of consciousness occur.

It is advisable to practice *Yoga Nidra* before actually going to sleep, because it's an excellent technique for inducing lucid dreaming and out-of-the-body experiences during sleep. Yoga masters remain aware even during deep sleep. Only the body and brain are fast asleep, whereas awareness is continuous.

During the practice, it is necessary to focus in quick succession on individual parts of the body. Mentally name each part feeling it as distinctly as possible. In the beginning, you may find it difficult to actually "feel" certain body parts. Don't let this worry you, but continue to rotate your awareness fairly rapidly.

The following is a description of the preliminary practice of *Yoga Nidra* for the purpose of increasing the power of the affirmations given in the practice of the five self-restraints:

- Lie flat on your back, with your arms stretched out by your sides, palms up.
- Place a pillow behind your neck for support and another pillow under your knees for added comfort.

- Take a couple of deep breaths, emphasizing the exhalation.
- Close your eyes. Repeat silently Om three times feeling the sound permeate the whole body.
- Form a clear intention – repeating a clear and prepared affirmation.
- Starting with your right side, rotate your awareness through all parts of the body - limb by limb - in fairly quick succession.
- Begin with the right thumb, first finger, second finger, ring finger, and little finger; feel the palm and then the back of the hand; the wrist, forearm, elbow, shoulder, arm-pit, right hip; thigh; knee; calf; ankles; top of the foot and then the bottom of the foot; right great toe, and each toe in succession.
- Repeat with the left side, starting with the left thumb, and ending with the left small toe.
- Now feel the right shoulder blade followed by the left shoulder blade, right small of the back, left small of the back, right buttock and left buttock in quick succession.
- Move to the right front chest, left front chest, right of the navel and left of the navel; right hip and left hip
- Feel the top of the head, front of forehead, right eye, left eye, right ear, left ear, nose, mouth, right cheek, left cheek, chin, right throat, left throat.
- Be aware of your body as a whole.
- Repeat the rotation one or more time to increase the depth of relaxation, always ending with whole-body awareness.
- Feel the navel and stay at this location while becoming aware of the breath; count down twelve slow breaths.
- Feel the front of the chest at the heart center, becoming aware of the breath; count down twelve slow breaths.
- Feel the front of the throat and become aware of the breath; count down twelve slow breaths.
- Repeat the affirmation.

- Prepare to return to ordinary consciousness, or turn over and go to sleep
- If you are returning to normal consciousness, gently move your fingers for a few moments, take a deep breath, and then open your eyes.

There is no time limit for the practice of *Yoga Nidra*, unless you impose one. So if you have things to do afterwards, make sure you set your wristwatch or clock for a gentle wakeup call.

Mudra

The Sanskrit word *mudra* means 'gesture' or 'attitude'. *Mudras* can be described as psychic, emotional, and devotional gestures or attitudes. *Yogis* have experienced *mudras* as attitudes of energy flow, intended to link individual *pranic* force with universal or cosmic force. The Kularnava Tantra traces the word *mudra* to the root *mud* meaning 'delight' or 'pleasure'. *Mudra* is also defined as a 'seal'.

Mudras are a combination of subtle physical movements which alter mood, attitude and perception, and which deepen awareness and concentration. A *mudra* may involve the whole body in a combination of *asana* (postures), *pranayama* (breath control), *bandha* (psycho-physical lock) and visualization techniques or it may be a simple hand position. The branch of *Hatha Yoga* treats *mudra* as an independent system of Yoga, requiring a very subtle awareness.

Mudras are usually only taught after some proficiency has been attained in *asana*, *pranayama* and *bandha*, and gross blockages have been removed. *Mudras* have been described in various texts from antiquity to the present day in order to preserve them for posterity. *Mudras* are higher practices which lead to awakening of the *prana* or life-force, *chakras* (energy centers) and *kundalini* (potential energy) and which can bestow major *siddhis* or psychic powers, on the advanced practitioner.

The attitudes and postures adopted during *mudra* practices establish a direct link between the Physical Body and the subtle body consisting of the Energy Body, Emotional Body, and Mental Body. A *mudra* establishes *pranic* balance within the *koshas* (bodies) and enables the redirection of subtle energy to the upper *chakras*, inducing higher states of consciousness. An analogy is much the same way that energy in the form of light or sound waves is diverted by a mirror. The *nadis* and *chakras* constantly radiate *prana* which normally escapes from the body and dissipates into the external world. By creating barriers within the body through the practice of *mudra*, the life-force energy is redirected within. For example, by closing the eyes with the fingers in *shanmukhi mudra*, the *prana* being radiated through the eyes is reflected back. In the same way, the sexual energy emitted through *vajra nadi* is redirected to the brain through the practice of *vajroli mudra*.

Once the dissipation of *prana* is arrested through the practice of *mudra*, the mind becomes introverted, inducing states of *pratyahara* or sense withdrawal and *dharana* (concentration). *Mudras* are of course important techniques for awakening *kundalini* because of their ability to re-direct *prana*. For this reason they are extensively incorporated in *Kriya* and *Kundalini* Yoga practices.

We are not going to delve into the *mudras* for awakening *kundalini*, but rather focus on certain hand *mudras* which are used for breaking up ingrained habit patterns of a negative nature. This is highlighted in the practice of the five restraints.

Japa

Japa is the mental or silent repetition of an aspect of divinity and is considered by saints and sages to be better than verbal repetition. With mental repetition, the mind is fixated, but in oral repetition the wandering mind may not be effectively stopped, unless it is absorbed in the sound.

If your mind wanders while chanting mentally or aloud, you will miss the joy that accompanies the one-pointedness of the mind on an aspect of the divine. Where one's love is, there one's mind is. Any object or person that you love with all your heart gives you great joy, just by the thought of it.

The goal of *japa* is to develop a steady and continuous consciousness of the divine. It is very powerful to fix oneself on the combinations of Sanskrit sounds called *mantra*. The *mantra* is an inherent, spiritual, mystical formula which has become "known" by a Self-Realized Yogi, who has then infused it with his life-force, and then transmitted it for the benefit of future generations of seekers of the truth. A *mantra* liberates the limited consciousness and helps us to cross over the sea of the uncontrolled and conditioned mind. It is not a good idea to give *mantras* in a book, as they should not be improperly pronounced and also there should be a legitimate transmission from a practitioner who has internalized the *mantra*.

The practice of *japa* can help us to maintain a continuous remembrance of the Divine – it is thinking of the Divine constantly, to the exclusion of everything else. Repetition of the Names of the Divine or *mantra* should be done with sincerity, faith, one-pointed concentration and devotion. It cannot be a mere robotic repetition - one of the critical ingredients is the power that we infuse into the word that produces the effect. When it is done with love and devotion, it sets up a vibration that keeps our mind and senses harmonized with the divine within us. With constant practice of *japa* one can transcend the mind and realize one's identity with the Divine.

If you have the good fortune to be initiated into a *mantra*, then its *japa* would be of great value in tuning into the divine aspect for the strength to practice the self-restraints. The *japa* is an effective part of the self-disciple of *ishvar pranidhan* or surrender to the Divine.

If you have not yet had the opportunity to obtain a *mantra*, then it is possible to substitute an English prayer, such as the Lord's Prayer.

Love

The most powerful tool for transformation is the power of Love. Even if you are not able to utilize any of the other tools or techniques, if you can harness this power, then spiritual transformation is assured.

We send life force or *prana* to whatever we give our attention to. Since our mind is always fluctuating, our attention waivers and the emotions are unsteady. The unsteady emotion called love is not the Love that needs to be cultivated. The emotional love is a commodity of exchange – it is bargained for implicitly or explicitly to obtain some sort of gratification. If one of two lovers suddenly fails to live up to their end of the bargain, that is, stop loving the one, then the other will be upset.

Love is unconditional, and is not a commodity of exchange. It exists at our deepest levels and is the state of our True Self – it is a state of the Divine within us.

When we understand how thoughts arise, we can then be better prepared to detach from them sufficiently that we can cultivate unconditional Love. All thoughts arise through the filter of the *samskaras*, or imprints of the consciousness. These *samskaras* are further combined to form *vasanas* or complex habit patterns. One's thoughts can arise through activating the *vasanas* by external sensory stimuli, such as something seen, or by memory, or by other external thought energy.

The first two sources for the thoughts should be quite familiar, but the third might need some clarification, for we are not always aware of how the thoughts of others can affect us. Our thoughts and therefore our emotions can be influenced by negative vibration contained in our environment. Thought energy in the form of vibration resonates with our subtle body, particularly the mental body and we pick up on negativity, anger or depression. Of course in a holy place and around holy people, we pick up positive and uplifting vibrations and our thoughts become more positive. The externally aroused thoughts resonate from the mental body down to the emotional body and the down to the energy body and lastly to the physical body by means of the nervous system. Our whole being becomes infected with the externally aroused thought patterns and resultant emotions.

Of course, if our subtle body does not have the resonant *samskaras* and *vasanas* to react to the external thoughts, then there will be no effect. However, only a Self-Realized Yogi will have be able to have purified the subtle body of all *samskaras*. For the rest of us, we should become more aware of the relationship between our habit patterns, the arising of thoughts, emotions and our actions.

Once we are aware that we are directing our life-force *prana* into those thought forms which we take ownership of, we can weaken this causal chain by the practice of detachment and unconditional Love. If thoughts become habitual and stimulate emotional responses, they become very powerful forces of creation. We create our own life, whether we realize it or not. If we think about Love and direct our energy into such thoughts, then it is projected and reflected in our lives.

However, if we let our thoughts and emotions, even those that do not come from us, build up until they get out of all proportion, and take over the whole of our awareness, then we lose the ability to cultivate Love. When we agree to identify with our emotions and find "we are angry," "we are depressed," or "we are afraid," then we allow ourselves to become lost in them. We get caught and bound up in the limitations of separateness and smallness. Be conscious of the feelings that come up, let them flow through, but detach from them. Become unlimited in the nobility and greatness of Love.

Cultivating positive thoughts and cheerful feelings have a purifying effect on the subtle body. The good news is that the subtle body is subject to the will and so a person can will himself to think positively and to feel good feelings. If the subtle body is impure, the thoughts and feelings will lack clarity, be negative, or be depressive in nature, while a more purified subtle body naturally is positive, and has more clarity – this is reflected in the quality of the thoughts..... it's like a feedback loop.... positive thoughts purify the subtle body and a more purified subtle body gives rise to more and more positive thoughts and less and less of negative thoughts!

Once the subtle body is gradually purified, you will be able to discern the underlying life-lessons to be learned in each of your negative thoughts and feelings. There are great opportunities for self-study in each negative emotion. It is said that when one truly lets go of all negative expressions of the mind, peace shines through, and Love becomes the only mode of one's expression.

It is a sober thought to reflect on the efforts many make to purify the physical body through the use of a variety of diets, but at the same time they totally neglect their subtle body. One's thoughts and feelings are food for one's subtle body, which will then reflect the thoughts and feelings it is fed. Cultivate positive thoughts and uplifting feelings today… and tomorrow.

By practicing the *yama* of truthfulness or *satya*, we will begin to see the One in all beings and things. When we begin to realize the underlying Reality, we begin to attain equanimity and freedom from selfish desires, and can then surrender our whole nature to the indwelling Spirit. In this way, pure Love arises. We attain freedom from acting by the forces of attraction and repulsion, friendship and enmity, pleasure and pain, when we are guided by Love and equanimity.

In the beginning the spiritual seeker should first try to remain centered in love, to remain loving under all circumstances. The heart center is the energy center which corresponds to our higher emotions and feelings – we should connect with the heart center and make it the conduit for our responding to the world around us. Feel from the heart and respond from the heart, not from the mind.

When you are absorbed in Love, the *manas* or mind is purified and you have accomplished the goal of all the five self-restraints of *yama*! When you are absorbed in Love, the subtle body is purified, and you have accomplished *saucha* (purity). When you are fully absorbed in Love, you realize that you are one with all beings, and one with the Divine, accomplishing the goal of *svadyaya* (self-study). When you are completely absorbed in Love, you are totally surrendered to the Divine, and have accomplished *ishvar pranidhana*.

Recommended helpful activities for cultivating Love:

- At least once a day, spend a little time on devotional chanting, and/or prayer.
- Maintain good personal hygiene and a tidy and clean living environment because one's external environment is a reflection of the internal subtle environment.
- Examine who you keep company with – avoid those who drain or depress you and seek out those who inspire you.
- Avoid speaking harshly to others – make your words helpful or keep silent.
- Once a week, keep a day of silence to recharge yourself and to purify your thoughts
- Let go of anger against anyone and do not entertain negative thoughts of others.

Practice for cultivating Love:

- Think of your spouse or a significant other or your best friend. Is there something about this person that irritates you? Recall that something, and let go of it; laugh about it. Then send your Love from your heart to this beloved person.
- Think of one of your parents. Recall all the sacrifices that your parent had to go through to raise you. Is there anything about your parent that you dislike? Let go of it. Then send you Love from your heart to this parent. (It is immaterial whether the parent is still on this physical plane.)
- Visualize your worst enemy. We all have someone whom we utterly detest, or who rubs us the wrong way, or who has done some really nasty things to us. Think of all the things that make you angry about this person – now, take a deep breath and let it all go with the exhale. You may have to repeat this several times before you feel that you have

given up the anger and hate associated with this person. Now send your Love to this person with a smile.

- Finally, think of the Divine aspect that you most identify with and feel yourself flooded with Love from the Divine.

It is recommended that one should do this practice at least once a week to detoxify ourselves from our negativity and to purify ourselves for the inflow of Divine Love.

Part 4
Practice:
Furthering Progress
on the
Path of Purification
&
Transformation

The Practice of Self-Restraint

Ahimsa: Non-harming, Nonviolence, Non-injury

In the state of divine union, *samadhi*, the *yogic* sages have unanimously stated that all life is one. If we are to achieve that realization, we must affirm that oneness and unity by being kind, compassionate and respectful to all living beings in thought, word and action.

We are advised to refrain from causing or wishing harm, distress or pain to any living being, including ourselves and the world we live in. It would also be necessary to dissuade others from harmful or violent actions - it is not enough to just avoid violence. We should not only refrain from violence against living beings, but in all its manifestations – there can be violence in the way you close a door, cut someone off on the freeway, or even call out a name.

Ahimsa is not merely non-killing or 'Thou shalt not kill'. To live in *ahimsa*, it is important to develop an attitude of perfect harmlessness with positive love and respect for all life, not just in our actions, but in our thoughts and words as well. With perfection of *ahimsa* one realizes the unity and oneness of all life and attains universal love, peace and harmony. With perfect practice of *ahimsa* one rises above anger, hatred, fear, envy and attachment.

Suggested practice of *ahimsa*:

1. We need to examine our personal life, work situations and social interactions, to observe how we can apply *ahimsa*. Next, visualize yourself at home, at work, and social situations, and imagine your reaction to certain challenges

to nonviolence. For example, what would you do, if your wife asks you to kill a spider on the wall? Or, if your husband wants you to punish your child?

2. Analyze your good and bad tendencies. Record in a journal, at the end of each day, your conduct, thoughts, words and actions. Be totally honest with yourself and make the necessary changes for improvement. Train your mind to think positive, inspiring thoughts.

3. Affirmation:

I will refrain from criticizing, fault-finding, judging and blaming others for mistakes. I consider myself and others worthy of love, forgiveness and respect. Love is my divine nature and I have an endless capacity for love, which is ever seeking expression through me. The Divine dwells within everyone's heart. All people are expressions of the One. There is no place for violence in love. There is no place for violence in life.

When you practice *Yoga Nidra*, as described in a previous section, the affirmation should be shortened for easy memorization as follows:

I'm completely filled with love and I express love to all beings under all situations.

4. Give service to others and perform all your actions with love and awareness, offering all the fruits of your action to the Divine. Forgive all those who have 'hurt' you.

5. Study the lives of great souls who have attained perfection in nonviolence, such as Buddha, Jesus Christ, Mahatma Gandhi, and Francis of Assisi.

6. Cultivate the positive traits recommended by those who have successfully perfected nonviolence:

- Focus on people's good points. Tell everyone with whom you come into contact the good things you see in them.
- Develop a positive approach toward life. Compliment more than you criticize.
- Build a climate of trust and support in all your relationships. Cooperate with others instead of competing with them.
- Use gentle, loving, and respectful language with everyone.
- Listen patiently, with your heart, when others are talking. Love means to put aside one's own interests for the love of another.
- Learn how to refuse with a smile. If you have to say "no" to something, do it respectfully.
- Don't put others down to make yourself look better.
- Never criticize others behind their back.
- Do extra little things that are nobody's job. Be generous by volunteering, especially for the jobs for which there is no great reward.
- Become an instrument of peace like the great sages - let us learn to tame what is wild and violent within ourselves and the world around us.

7. Color is the visible vibrations of light energy. All light emanates from the sun, the great ocean of light and the source of all life. The Seven Rays are of the visible spectrum: red, orange, yellow, green, blue, indigo and violet. Not only the physical world but also the energetic, emotional, mental and spiritual planes are sustained by the

Sun's White Light. From an individual's point of view, this means that color affects us physically, energetically, emotionally, mentally, and spiritually. Our thoughts and feelings vibrate to color and to the fields around our five bodies, which some label the auras, continuously throwing out all manners of colors.

Why does one person prefer certain colors and are repelled by others? All matter radiates light and has a color vibration, which is continuously emitted and has an affect based on the reaction from the "color consciousness" of the person.

The "color consciousness" is the aggregate of the "color state" of the energy centers or *chakras*. This "color state" is a complex of the balance and health of the energy centers.

The color blue is particularly suitable for the practice of *ahimsa*. Visualize the blue color in a round ball for about five minute to induce a calm state of mind. Surround yourself with blue objects or wear blue clothing. The shade of blue should be quite deep but not dark, nor pastel, for the optimum effect.

8. *Mudra* for Gentleness:
   Sit comfortably with the back straight. Grasp the thumb of each hand in a fist and bring the fists to each side of the temple, with the wrists at about eye level. The elbows are facing outward toward the front. Press the fists gently on the head. Close your eyes, and breathe deeply for a minute and then keeping the wrist still on the temple, spread the fingers of each hand. Open your eyes and breathe deeply for a minute. Close the fists again and close your eyes for another minute.

9. *Mudra* for Courage:

   Sit comfortably with the back straight. Bend the left arm at the elbow and hold your hand a few inches in front of the navel, with the palm facing up. Lift the right arm and hold the hand in front of the right shoulder with the palm turned outward towards the front, fingers pointing upward. Focus your eyes on the mid-point between the eye-brows, with eyes half-open. Breathe deeply and slowly for about five minutes.

Satya: *Non-lying, Truthfulness*

Truth or *Sat* is one of the aspects of the Divine. As our essential nature is this same Divinity, it is against our true nature to exaggerate, pretend, distort or lie to others, or to manipulate people for our own selfish concerns. When we live in truthfulness we become anchored in the awareness of the Divine.

Why do we lie? It is because of selfishness and the fear of losing one's reputation. However, you can fool some of the people some of the time, but you can never fool your true Self anytime! Honesty with oneself is the first step towards self-improvement.

Can someone achieve any self-realization or self-knowledge by lying to others and to oneself? If you tell lies, you build up a false personality, which consists of lies and you deceive yourself. If you are immersed in lying, you will never know the truth or the Divine.

There is a story from the life of King Harishchandra which provides a very good example of a man devoted to *satya*. Harischandra was the king of Ayodhya in an age before Rama. He was a just and wise ruler and his kingdom prospered under him, which made him very proud.

One day he heard that the *rishi* Vishvamitra was passing through his lands, and he hastily went out to meet with the great sage. The king paid his respects to the sage and asked him to bless his palace with his presence, as he wanted to take the sage as his preceptor. Vishvamitra knew that the king was not yet ready to take a Guru, and declined. However, the king persisted, and the sage decided to test his sincerity by asking for huge amount as a *Guru-dakshina*, or offering to the preceptor.

The proud king agreed. Moreover, he knelt before the sage and offered his whole kingdom and all its wealth at the feet of

Vishvamitra, who accepted the offering. However, much to the shock of the king, the sage still insisted on receiving the *Guru-dakshina*. Since the Harishchandra had already offered everything he had to his intended Master, he had nothing left to make up the offering required.

Being a man of his word, he could not take back what he had promised, and so said, "Give me a month's time and I shall give you that too."

He then proceeded with his wife and son to leave his lands, dressed only in the most humble of clothing. The royal family then proceeded towards Kashi. Arriving there, Harishchandra sought work but could find none. They were forced to beg for a living. A month passed, and the sage again appeared before Harishchandra, and pressed him for the offering.

Seeing her husband's plight, the queen insisted, "Sell me as a slave, my lord, and fulfill your promise." Reluctantly, Harishchandra agreed. He sold his wife and even his son, but still couldn't raise the required gold coins. He then sold himself and was finally able to fulfill his promise to the sage. The queen and the prince had to toil long hours for a merchant. Still the merchant remained unsatisfied, Meanwhile, Harishchandra's master appointed him as an assistant in the cremation fields, the lowliest and most dishonorable role imaginable.

After a year had passed, one fateful day Harishchandra's son was bitten by a snake and died. The heart broken mother carried the dead child to the cremation field. The former king was shattered to see his wife bearing the dead body of their child. Still, he had to do his duty! "I am sorry, my dear," he said tearfully, "I cannot cremate our son unless you pay the cremation fees required by my master." "My Lord, I am a penniless slave," cried his wife. In despair the couple decided to kill themselves in the funeral pyre with their son. After Harishchandra made a pyre of half burnt logs, and placed their dead child on it, they, seating themselves besides their child, ready to set the pyre ablaze.

At that moment Vishvamitra appeared and blessed them, bringing the prince back to life and restoring the crown to Harishchandra. The sage smiled and told him, "you have proved beyond doubt that you are the most honest man on earth. Your trials are over. Your son will now rule the kingdom and you and your wife can go to a heavenly abode."

When one who is established in truth prays with a pure heart, then things he really need come to him when they are really needed, he does not have to run after them. The man firmly established in truth gets the fruit of his actions without apparently doing anything. God, the source of all truth, supplies his needs and looks after his welfare.

Truth should not be used to hurt or harm another – it should be used compassionately with *ahimsa* in mind. To be truthful is not to be tactless. Thoughtfulness is essential to the usefulness of truth in relationship to others.

By thinking, speaking and acting in truth you will have peace of mind, free from fear, anxiety and worry. You will be respected by people from all walks of life. The power of the universe is harnessed in the thoughts, words and deeds of those who live in truth.

On a higher level, *satya* is the truth of our essential nature, which as Shri Yukteswar, the great *Kriya* Master says:

> *Man is a soul and has a body. When he properly places his sense of identity, he leaves behind all compulsive patterns. So long as he remains confused in his ordinary*

state of spiritual amnesia, he will know the subtle fetters of environmental law.

In this context, the supreme truth is the self-knowledge which reveals the world as it is. By constant contemplation of the supreme truth, enlightenment is attained. Self-study or *svadhyaya*, one of the *niyama* is impossible to practice without the fundamental development of *satya*.

The Practice of *Satya*

1. Practice a period of silence, at least once a week, and tune in to the Divine aspect of Truth in the stillness of silence. During this period of silence, remain in a state of mindful awareness. To be still is to be in the presence of Divine - listen to Psalm 46:10 as it says: "Be still and know that I am God." By understanding this simple verse we begin to find inner communion with the Divine, which speaks to our minds, fills our hearts with truth and inspiration when our consciousness is attuned to the inner silence. When the mind is silent, energy slowly gathers. Thought and egotistic preoccupations scatter the energy. When the mind is still, it reflects life accurately, without distortion.

2. Use *Yoga Nidra* to so that introspection and self-observation can take place when the mind is still and becomes aware of the different types of thoughts, desires, longings and fears. Observe every thought and feeling as it arises in the mind, being aware of its cause, content and meaning. By observing your thoughts like this, suppressed experiences in the unconscious mind start to unfold themselves. Tremendous energy is released while unburdening the unconscious mind of all conflict. After some time of practice the mind will experience a stillness in which there is no observer or

observed. Awareness of silence and peace is stabilized in truth, as delusions and illusions of the mind are forsaken.

2. **Affirmation**

I am committed to express truth in my live as a means to self-realization, as a blessing to every person I meet, without hurt or harm. I express truth in thought, word and deed to all living beings. I live in truth, love and harmony, and share it with others.

With *Yoga Nidra*, use the following shortened affirmation:

I express truth in thought, word and deed to all living beings, under the guidance of Love.

3. Be aware of your thoughts, when you interact at home, in the office or social activities. Only speak those words which are truthful. Before you speak, examine your thoughts to determine if they are selfish or harmful. Will they cause distress to someone? Your thoughts, words and actions should be in harmony with each other and to truth.

4. Understand yourself. Be ready to admit your faults and errors without feelings of guilt or sorrow - it is the first step to self improvement. Search out truths about yourself on all levels, including your likes and dislikes, without being judgemental or prejudiced.

5. Develop an attitude of truthfulness. Always recognize and accept the state of things and circumstances as they are and work with what is.

6. Visualize yourself in different situations where truth is an issue, and analyze your possible reactions, in the light of

the Divine. Will you tell a lie to save someone from death? What about lying to ensure a murderer is put away from harming others? We shall examine such potentially conflicting moral issues in the last section of the book, but it will be helpful if you think about it before reading that section.

7. Visualize the color violet as a long egg-shape surrounding your body. Do this for five minutes, whenever you feel yourself disconnected from the principle of truth.

8. *Mudra*:
   Form with your left hand the *jnana mudra* or gesture of wisdom, by touching the tip of the index finger to the edge of the thumb, forming roughly a square.

   Form your right hand in the *chin mudra* or gesture of control, by touching the tip of the index finger to the tip of the thumb and forming a circle.

   Place both hands on the thighs, without tension and hold for about five minutes. Keep your back straight. This is the *mudra* which connects to the Universal Principle of Truth within oneself.

Asteya: Non-stealing

The primary cause for people stealing is the lack of contentment, which leads to greed and desire, manifesting as insecurity, selfishness and poverty consciousness.

When we are discontent with the present, desire keeps one continually looking to the future for one's fulfillment, instead of realizing that perfection is attainable here and now. To try to gain satisfaction by fulfilling the endless desires that arise in the mind is an utterly futile endeavor which only causes unhappiness and sorrow. We all know this in our hearts, but our minds choose to ignore the wisdom of our souls.

Desire arises from the ego or "I" consciousness, from the thoughts of 'I want', 'I need', or 'I must have'. In the experience of the great sages, contentment arises only from permanent happiness and joy, permanent peace, and love, and not in the satisfaction of passing desires. To experience this we must look within and discover that true and permanent happiness cannot be found outside of ourselves.

The mind is constantly turning outward, because it believes that fulfillment lies in the external world. However, like all the other great *yogis*, Jesus had taught: "The Kingdom of God is within you." (Luke 17:2), and, once you attain love, joy and peace from within, it will also come to you from without.

Just as we forget our "I" during deep sleep, we forget our true Self or Identity to the Divine, during our waking state. It is through this forgetfulness of our true identity and our relationship to the Divine that we feel lost, experience unhappiness and live in poverty consciousness. Until we have a conscious awareness of the Divine's presence within, it cannot bear fruit in our experience.

Once we are attuned and surrendered to the Divine, we become consciously aware, and open to the universe, which provides all that we need. We derive everything from Divine Consciousness and we are all a part of the One Consciousness.

You must eliminate all negative thoughts of lack, poverty and failure from your mind. Live from within by attuning your will with the Divine Will, and let Divine Wisdom be your guide in everything. Stealing shows a distrust of the intimate relationship with the Divine. We must realize that every breath we take is by Divine grace. The Divine is the source and cause of all. The Divine rained Manna from the skies to feed the hungry people because Moses trusted in the Divine.

Is it right to steal a loaf of bread to feed a dying child? We can always rationalize or justify certain actions, but even such a kind action is a transgression that has to be held accountable. Of course, it may be balanced on the scales of *karma*, by the compassion of saving a life, and yet it is a consequence of a lesser consciousness. In higher consciousness and trust in the Divine, the Divine compassion will supply the child with food somehow.

It is not only material objects which can be stolen, but stealing can also occur on a subtle level, by the stealing people's time, affections, emotions, attention, ideas and thoughts. There are some who perform these acts of subtle stealing consciously, while others do them subconsciously, out of a need to win attention and fame for themselves.

It is also important to realize that stealing can cause the breaking of other *yamas*. If we try to conceal a theft, we would lie, or even resort to violence against another living being.

Also, *asteya* includes misappropriation, breach of trust, mismanagement and misuse. The epic Ramayana provides a good example of a man who devotedly practiced the principle of *asteya*. His name was Prince Bharat, whose father, King Dasaratha, was the ruler of Ayodhya, and whose elder brother was Crown Prince Rama.

Dasaratha had three wives. The middle wife Kaikeyi was the mother of Prince Bharata. Once while Prince Bharata was away at his grandfather's house his mother learned that Prince Rama was to be crowned the king soon. This upset her. She went to her husband and said, "Grant me the two boons you had promised me years ago." "Certainly my beloved," replied the King. "First," said the ambitious Kaikeyi, "Let my son Bharata be crowned king and second, banish Rama to the forest for fourteen years."

King Dasaratha was heart-broken at Kaikeyi's cruel demands. However, he was bound by his promise and granted Kaikeyi her boons. The obedient prince Rama left for the forest accompanied by his wife, Sita, and brother, Lakshmana. Urgent summons were sent to Prince Bharata to return. Meanwhile, the aged King Dasaratha died of grief.

As Bharata entered Ayodhya he noticed the down-cast faces of the people. "Something is seriously wrong," he thought to himself as he rushed to his mother's chamber. Kaikeyi was delighted to see her son. "Oh Bharata," she exclaimed, you shall be crowned the king of Ayodhya! Your father is no more, and I have had Rama banished to the forest for fourteen years.

The righteous Bharata was horrified at his mother's words. "Oh, Mother", he cried, "You have been blinded by greed.! I have no use for power, nor do I wish to rob my brother, Rama, of his kingdom!" Bharata immediately left for the forest. "I must bring my beloved brother Rama back to rule his kingdom," he resolved.

In the forest Bharata met up with Rama, and falling at his feet, the pure-hearted Bharata sobbed, asked for forgiveness and proclaimed his innocence. "Please return to govern your land and people. Our father, the king is no more". Rama knew that Bharata was faultless, but he could not be persuaded to come out of exile, because he would obey his father's last command.

However, he agreed to return to rule if Bharata would serve as the king during his absence.

Bharata reluctantly agreed, but before departing, he begged Rama to give him his sandals. On returning to Ayodhya, Bharata humbly placed Rama's sandals on the throne. He then moved to a hermitage on the outskirts of Ayodhya. Living the simple life of an ascetic he ruled the kingdom from there. When Rama returned from exile after fourteen years, the pure-hearted Bharata gladly handed over the kingdom to Lord Rama.

The Practice of *Asteya*

1. Channel all your desires into one desire – the desire for Self-realization. Realize and understand that it is the desire or need for something apart from the Divine that keeps us separate from the Universal Source of All.

   It is false to believe that we can be satisfied with something outside of ourselves, other than the presence and the Power of the Divine.

   When you hold the desire for union with the Divine, that is Yoga, above all other desires, then they will subside.

2. Develop a consciousness of abundance, and you will receive freely from the universal supply. Attune your will to the Divine Will. Realize that if you have any sense of lack, it is

because your thoughts, ideas and beliefs have conditioned your mind to hold these limitations. Turn your thoughts from lack and limitation to the belief in the inevitable operation of the Divine Giver working for you in abundance.

3. Think about your ideal – the way you want to be based on what you've learned about yourself so far. Visualize yourself as you want to be. Retain that image and sustain it joyfully with faith and expectancy until you succeed in its attainment. Do this regularly.

4. Examine your life and relationships and eliminate all non-essential things and activities.

   You may wish to consider minimizing your contacts with egocentric people who have conflicting and negative patterns of thought to your spiritual views on life.

5. Practice *Karma Yoga* by giving service to others, with no expectation of reward.

   This awakens compassion and takes attention away from our own personal feelings of lack. When we consciously serve and give from our heart, we attract the down-flow of Divine grace into our lives.

6. **Affirmation**

   The Divine is infinite abundance, and I am an individualized expression of Divinity. My birthright is the ceaseless flow of abundance, love, peace, joy, health, power and energy. I have everything I need, because the Divine is manifested within my consciousness and the Divine is the only source of all. By taking responsibility for my thoughts, words and deeds, and acting in accordance with the principles of self-restraint, I am ever moving towards Self-realization.

When practiced together with *Yoga Nidra*, use the abbreviated form of the affirmation:

I am happy and content for I lack nothing. Ever filled with abundance, I'm a giver and not a taker.

Brahmacharya: Non-sensuality, Conservation of Energy

Brahmacharya is consciousness that is anchored in the Divine. It is mind ever turned towards the Divine. It is the state of Yoga or ecstatic union with the Source of All. In this state of Yoga, *brahmacharya* becomes effortless. However, while on the path until Yoga is achieved, continuous effort is necessary to turn our thoughts, words and actions towards the Divine.

In ancient India, most saints and *yogis* were householders. They would bring up families, performing their duties to society, while continuing their practice of Yoga and leading a spiritual life. To them, there was no conflict between sex and God. Asceticism and celibacy were temporary periods of intense practice, but not necessarily a way of life, until monastic Buddhism entered into the Indian religious tradition. It is instructive to remember that the Buddha married and had a son prior to taking up the ascetic path.

Nowadays, most people are interpreting *brahmacharya* as only meaning the restraint of the sex impulses or celibacy, rather than as a sublimation of all passions through deeper emotions of loving kindness and affection. If *brahmacharya* only meant celibacy then married people who wanted children would not be able to practice Yoga. It is because *brahmacharya* has a wider meaning than the restraint of the sexual impulse, that there have been so many householder saints with children. The greatest *yogis* and *rishis* of all times, such as Vashista and Yagnavalkya were householders, and in recent times, there was Lahiri Mahasaya who, in 1861, was initiated into the ancient techniques of Kriya Yoga in the Himalayas, by the immortal master Mahavatar Babaji. Lahiri Mahasaya and his wife had five children born to them, some years after Lahiri's initiation by Babaji.

Sexuality is regarded as an obstacle to spiritual life, in the Judeo-Christian religions and this has falsely programmed negative feelings of guilt, shame and sin, in the modern consciousness, towards something the Divine has created for the purposes of procreation and creativity.

Although *brahmacharya* should be practiced at all levels of energy usage, it is necessary that in these days, where sexual excitation is rampant in all walks of life, and sexual frustration is at all time highs, we should first examine the sexual perspective above all others.

From a spiritual or moral point of view, a sexual relationship should be based on commitment. There has to be commitment and loving concern for each other to make the relationship meaningful. Sexuality is not just a toy provided for our physical pleasures divorced from responsibility and care. A relationship for the purpose of possessing an object for ego-gratification through the senses is meaningless. For a true relationship to form, the identification of others as objects for self-gratification must end. Love can express itself naturally and spontaneously in joyful sexual intimacy without feelings of guilt or shame. However, if a relationship is based on self-gratification, it will eventually be destroyed by the ill-feelings of the partner who is being disregarded.

Therefore *brahmacharya* is not the abandonment of sex, but its placement in a spiritual perspective. The question is not, 'Shall I renounce sex, marriage and social responsibility for a life of spiritual practice?' but 'What is my right relationship to them?' It is the same question, whether one is following the householder's path or the path of renunciation.

Some are attached to sexual indulgence, making sex into an addiction, as they strive towards ever more and stronger orgasms. The mind becomes obsessed with sex, causing undue tension.

Excessive indulgence in sexuality leads to sorrow and pain. The mind is agitated, while the intellect is impaired and unable to discriminate. Physical radiance and magnetism decreases with lose of sexual energy and vitality. Boredom, depression and discontent sets in, as in all obsessions and addictions.

On the other hand, repression or denial can be just as harmful as indulgence – both are be ego-centric, and makes the mind dull, losing its sensitivity and awareness. There is no lasting joy in either indulgence or repression. Monastics and priests who try to deny their sexual natures, without the proper perspective, and methods of practice, eventually harm themselves and others as they secretly try to gratify their perverted, rather than sublimated natures. This is amply demonstrated by the recent scandals involving so-called 'celibate' priests of different religious persuasions.

Brahmacharya is the highest form of self-control. When one is established in *brahmacharya*, one develops an infinite source of vitality and energy, a courageous mind and a powerful intellect so that one can fight any type of injustice. The *brahmachari* will use the forces he generates wisely - he will utilize the physical ones for doing the work of the Lord, the mental for the spread of culture and the intellectual for the growth of spiritual life.

An example of a great *brahmacharya* was Shuka, the son of Sage Vyasa. As a young boy, he had been sent to study under another sage. Shuka was a keen and intelligent student and mastered everything he was taught. When Shuka returned home he continued to study and practice Yoga. A few years passed, and still Shuka kept his *brahmacharya* vows. However, his father Vyasa thought, "Shuka is now a young man. It is time for him to marry." When Vyasa proposed that Shuka get married, the young man replied that he wanted to remain a renunciate for the attainment of salvation.

The learned sage continued to teach his son many further philosophical scriptures. Still, Shuka thirsted for knowledge. Vyasa then advised his son, "Seek out Janaka, the king of Mithila, and study under him. He is the wisest man on earth." Shuka set off for the distant kingdom, journeying over mountains and through forests for two years. Finally, he arrived at Janaka's palace. Through his yogic powers, King Janaka already knew of Shuka's arrival and the purpose of his visit, but decided to test Shuka - he instructed the sentries not to honor or welcome the young man at the palace gates. Shuka was made to wait for three days. He waited patiently, undisturbed by this unkind reception.

On the fourth day Janaka arrived at the gates, welcoming Shuka and led him to the guest room. There Shuka was provided with every comfort. He was bathed and perfumed in water, dressed in silken robes and given delicious food. Shuka showed no greed or great delight at these luxuries. Instead he spent his days in meditation and prayer.

Because neither insults nor luxuries affected Shuka, King Janaka decided to put him to one final test. In the splendid court room filled with dazzling naked beauties, King Janaka gave Shuka a bowl full of milk, and said to him, "make seven rounds of this hall without spilling one drop of milk." Shuka accepted the bowl. He walked effortlessly around the great hall seven times, past the naked dancing and whirling ladies, without spilling a single drop of milk.

King Janaka was delighted. "Shuka," he said, "You are unequalled in your self-control and self-discipline. I have nothing further to teach you. Continue your practices and you will attain the supreme enlightenment."

The Practice of *Brahmacharya*

It is instructive to remember the words of Krishna, in counseling moderation in all things:

> *Yoga is not for those who eat too much, or too little, nor for those who sleep too much or too little. It is for those who are moderate in eating, sleeping, wakefulness, recreation and all actions, that yoga will bring an end to all sorrows. Those who have learned to discipline their minds and remain calmly established in the Self, free from attachment to all desires, attain to the state of union.*

1. Meditate on Desire.

One should ask oneself, 'Where do my desires come from? Did this desire come from the egoic 'I' or from my true Self? Why has this thought or desire entered my mind? Whom does it concern? Who is the 'I' who desires? What is the relationship between my true Self and this desire?

Only by understanding the nature of desires can you prevent them. By turning the mind inward to investigate its own source and nature, it is illuminated by the Self. If you practice this Self-enquiry constantly and persistently, eventually all other thoughts will drop away, and the ego will disappear.

When the mind is turned outward and lost in desires and attachments, our true eternal nature, is forgotten. We forget our true Self through identification with the body, mind and ego. We experience happiness and unhappiness, pleasure and pain because the body and mind are not permanent and subject to change. Treasured possessions are lost, and we cannot even hold on to the temporary states of joy that occur in our lives. That which changes cannot be real, only that which is permanent and eternal is real. **Remember that we are a soul with a body and not a body with a soul.**

Meditate on these words from Lord Krishna:

From thought comes attachment. From attachment desire arises. When desire is frustrated by an obstacle, anger springs up

When there is anger, one becomes easily deluded and loses memory of right and wrong. Loss of memory then leads to loss of discrimination. From this loss of intelligence, spiritual life is wasted.

But those who can supervise the involvement between the senses and sense-objects by exercising self-control and who become free thereby from craving and from false repression attain inner calmness, in which all sorrows end. Then one soon becomes established in the Self.
Bhagavad Gita (2:62-5)

When one is calmly centered within, in a state of attentive awareness at all times, free from conflict, then energy is conserved.

2. Transformation of sexual energy.

Practice regular meditation to overcome egocentric thoughts and emotions, and to hold everyone in respect as of equally divine nature. Such meditation will turn the energy inwards and upwards to higher centers of awareness.

The proper practice of Yoga and meditation transforms the sexual energy (semen or ovum on the physical level) into spiritual or subtle energy (*ojas*) by directing and channeling it upwards towards the higher energy centers, or *chakras*, through the subtle pathway in the spine called the *sushmna nadi*.

When you are following a spiritual path and are not married or in a sexual relationship, you will find Yoga postures and practices helpful in conserving and transforming the sexual energy on the physical level into *ojas* on the spiritual level.

Men lose more of the vital fluid during the sexual act than the women do, but both have vital fluids whose loss due to excessive sexual indulgence causes loss of vitality and unsteadiness of life-force *prana* in the body. Those people who are married or in a sexual relationship will benefit from these practices, as they have rejuvenating and toning effects on the sex centers, glands, nerves, and body systems, promoting longevity and vitality.

A series of *Hatha Yoga* exercises which are very helpful in the transformation of sexual energy are the *bandhas*. These are the muscular locks which are activated by constricting and relaxing certain muscles. They are sometimes practiced with holding of breath in certain breathing techniques, but for our purposes, we recommend that there is no holding of breath during the practice of the *bandhas*.

There three *bandhas* which are activated in a sequence to transform the sexual energy to spiritual energy. They should be practiced with the back straight, while sitting on the floor or at the edge of a chair.

First, we activate the root lock, called the *mulabandha*. This is done by constricting the external and internal sphincter muscles or the anal area. Specifically, first the muscles of the perineum [area between the anus and the genitals] are lightly contracted, followed by the closing of the anal muscles with moderate force. You will feel an upward pressure. Hold this contraction for about three minutes, continuing to breathe normally. Relax the muscles for about thirty seconds.

Next, contract the abdominal muscles at the navel, pulling in the abdomen as far back as possible without strain. Keep breathing and hold this contraction for about three minutes. Relax for about thirty seconds.

Then, raise your shoulders and lower your head so that that chin touches the hollow at the throat. Hold this with normal breathing for about three minutes. Focus on the space between the eyebrows, with eyes closed. Then relax for thirty seconds.

Finally, perform all three locks. Contract the muscles of the perineum and anal sphincter, followed by pulling in the navel, and lowering of the head. Focus all your attention on the third-eye center, the space above and behind the eye-brows. Feel energy moving from the perineum to the third-eye. Hold this for about three minutes, with normal breathing.

These locks are very powerful life-changing techniques and should be practiced carefully and in moderation.

3. Affirmation

I open myself to the inflow of Divine grace – it is Divine Wisdom which guides me towards true joy and inspires me to right thoughts, speech and actions. I use my energy wisely neither pursuing excess sensuality, nor repressing my sexual nature. My sexual energy is channeled into true love and positive attitudes. My mind is ever turned towards the Divine.

During *Yoga Nidra*, use the following abbreviated affirmation:

I channel my energies including sexual energy towards the Divine and express them in love and positive attitudes.

Aparigraha: Non-attachment, Non-greed

The Sanskrit word *apara* means 'of another' and *agraha* means 'to crave for'. Therefore, *aparigraha* is usually translated as 'without craving for that which belongs to another.' However, in a deeper sense, it means not to be craving for the "unreal", the "not-self" – it is non-attachment to everything that is not the True Self.

Non-greed, in this context, is not only resisting the temptation to covet what belongs to others, but also means non-attachment even to one's own possessions, as well as not to hoard or accumulate unnecessary amounts of something.

Unsteadiness of the mind or restlessness is an obstacle to spiritual progress. In his Yoga Sutras (2:3), *Patanjali* lists five afflictions that disturb mental equilibrium: ignorance, egoism, attraction to pleasure and aversion to pain, and clinging to life. Of these five afflictions, ignorance (*avidya*) is the source of all the other obstacles.

Ignorance leads to a mistaken sense of duality, which gives rise to a desire to experience, from which egoism or "I-sense" takes root. The ego principle gives rise to greed and insecurity.

Lord Krishna has given the following assurance:

> *To those who worship Me alone, and constantly meditate on Me, without any other thought, I provide all their needs and give full security.*
> *Bhagavad Gita, 9:22*

We receive Divine Grace in greater abundance, when we open and attune ourselves to the Divine Will. With faith in, and understanding of, Divine Grace, one can live a more fulfilling life.

Greed arises when the mind clings to the mistaken belief concerning where one's security is derived from - 'I will die without that person!', 'My security comes from being in this job, owning this house and being with my family.' In this way, we develop a false basis for our security by placing our power in such transitory things or by accumulating more possessions than we actually need.

When we act from attachment, we try to manipulate situations and other people, out of fear of losing the desired object. Subjected to selfish desires, fear and greed, one lives an insecure life.

It is instructive to remind ourselves that, **we come into this world with nothing, and we depart with nothing.**

However, let us not make the mistake of thinking that *aparigraha* is about giving up the possessions or wealth which can be useful in a limited way. It is about being unattached to them. In this context, there is the story of King Janaka, a Rajarishi:

King Janaka of Mithila was a disciple of sage Yajnavalkya. Though a king, he was totally detached in his attitude to kingship and his treasures. He was hailed as a *Raja-Rishi*, a sage and a king simultaneously. He performed his royal duties conscientiously and perfectly. However, he ensured that he did not develop any semblance of attachment towards anything attached to his regal position.

As the disciple was also a true and worthwhile seeker of spiritual knowledge, the preceptor went very much out of his way to impart all the sacred knowledge to him. However, this was mistaken by the other disciples who naturally thought that Janaka was being shown special preference only because of his royal status. In their opinion, Janaka was no better than any of them in spiritual matters.

Once, the king was late, but the sage decided to wait for his arrival before starting his *satsang* or spiritual instruction. The other disciples were upset and restless. Yajnavalkya knew what they were thinking and he wanted to educate them properly. The sincerity and impartiality of the preceptor should never be doubted by his disciples. This was the lesson he wanted to impart to his disciples.

After Janaka had arrived and paid his respects to the Master, the sage started his instruction. Soon the other disciples noticed that there was smoke in the distance where the city was and became a little worried. After a very short time, a messenger rushed in, approached king Janaka and told him in a distressed voice that Mithila was on fire and the king's palace, his family and friends, and all his possessions were in serious danger. King Janaka was unfazed and unmoved. He was not at all upset by this news of terrible catastrophe and impending doom. He told the messenger that he was engaged in spiritual matters with his preceptor and should not be disturbed over minor matters!

The rest of the disciples, however, were quite disturbed – some who were from the city were worried about their family and possessions, while others were worried that the raging fire would spread to their hermitage. They rushed out without, some going towards the city while others just milled around in their distress.

Sage Yajnavalkya and *sishya* Janaka continued their discussions. Soon the disciples returned and covered their faces with shame as they reported to their Guru that there was no fire at all, and it was only an illusion. They had realized that this illusion of a fire must have been created by their preceptor to test them. They had shown meaningless attachment to their small possessions while king Janaka had shown non-attachment to his palaces and treasures.

When Janaka was queried about his equanimity in the face of apparent disaster he replied calmly, "Nothing belongs to me really.

If there were fire, my ministers and attendants would have taken proper steps to extinguish it. What could I have done alone? I have no attachment to anything. I have faith in my officials. It is not as if I have abdicated my responsibilities. There is no way my kingdom could have caught fire so rapidly, so disastrously, without a cause too. The State is well protected. I did not trouble myself, therefore."

The Master looked at his disciples with a smile and they hung their heads in shame!

Our true security is in the Divine, which is always with us, within our hearts. When you let the Divine move into every area of your life, the spirit of truth and love becomes the foundation of your security.

The Practice of *Aparigraha*

1. **Meditate on greed.**
   Begin by analyzing the aspects of greed.
   One should meditate as follows:
   Think of something that you really like or want at this moment. Why do you want it? Can you live without it? How much of it do you need? As you continue in this way, repeat with other objects of desire and greed. In this way, the heart is purified.

2. Visualize yourself getting unlimited amounts of what you crave for. This can be elaborated as you spend time imagining yourself enjoying and reveling in the midst of your desired possessions. How do you feel? Are you satisfied? Do you want more? Are your sure you won't lose everything? Are other people going to steal from you? Are you worried or scared?

   Now see yourself stripped of everything that you have? How do you feel now?

3. Meditate regularly to cleanse your subconscious mind of the attachment to objects and persons.

    Release attachment to objects, relationships, bad habits, negative attitudes and conditionings which block your experience of truth. Let Divine Wisdom and grace be your guide, and strength.

    When there is hatred, resentment, anger, jealousy or violence toward another, the mind and breath become unsteady. Abandon all destructive and negative thoughts - cultivate the opposite, positive qualities of love, compassion, patience, tolerance, and kindness.

4. There are two *pranayama* techniques which work together to calm the unsteady mind:

    Take a slow deep breath through the nose and feel your whole body filled with this breath, barely holding the breath for a second or two. Then look to the left, and exhale forcefully with your mouth, feeling all negativity being expelled with the breath. Repeat two more times.

    Then, practice equal breathing with both nostrils – equalizing the inhalation and exhalation. This is very calming and energizing – it takes only a little effort to count the duration of inhalation and make the exhalation to the same count. When you are agitated, practice this equal breathing to let go of the negative state. In this way, you cultivate equanimity and calmness.

5. Affirmation

    I release all negative attitudes and conditionings which hinder my spiritual progress and accept life and whatever the Divine gives me. I know that I am never alone – the Divine is always with me and is the source of strength, freedom and security. I release all attachments to actions and the results of actions. The Divine Giver gives constantly and continuously and the love that I give is an expression of the Divine Love.

With *Yoga Nidra*, use the short version of the affirmation:

I am free from all attachments to my body, mind and senses, and to all possessions and relationships. I am now free to love unconditionally.

Overcoming Obstacles in the Practice of Self-Discipline

Self-Discipline requires constant Self awareness, which in turn always involves the removal of obstacles and obstructions from the body and mind. As these obstructions which cloud our understanding with ignorance and misunderstanding are wiped away, the inner joy and light of the Self that is ever-existent can shine in perfect Self-awareness.

There are many obstacles to the practicing of self-discipline and the sage Patanjali has enumerated the nine major ones as follows:

> *Disease, dullness, doubt, carelessness, laziness, sensuality, false perception, failure to reach firm ground and instability – these distractions of consciousness are obstacles.*
> *Yoga Sutras 1.30*

There are four symptoms which help the practitioner know that one or more of the nine obstacles are in affect:

> *Mental pain, despair, nervousness and irregular breathing are the symptoms of a distracted state of mind.*
> *Yoga Sutras 1.31*

There is a need for constant vigilance against falling into one of the negative mental states, and awareness is the most useful too for this purpose. When you feel pain or sorrow, the mind becomes distracted from that True Self, which is beyond pain. Meditation is difficult when the mind is distracted by painful memories or emotional hurts. Pain can be eliminated by examining it and letting it go – who is the experiencing the pain? How do this "I" arise? Why doesn't this "I" arise in sleep? Am "I" really in pain?

Despair is a mind being distracted by negative moods, frustration and anxiety. Moods are the result of low or negative energy. Change the energy level and its direction and you will develop a positive state of mind. You can overcome a mood with the following practice through regular exercise and finding something interesting to do.

It is relatively easy to identify nervousness when it is happening to someone else. However, when one is suffering from it, there may be some denial! In the extreme, when the body is restless, twitching and itching, it is difficult to focus your attention in meditation. The regular practice of Yoga postures or *asanas* can help the body become more steady.

Uneven inhalation and exhalation is caused by fluctuations of the mind and emotional instability. Since the mind and breath are yoked together, ff you are attentive to your breathing, you will be aware of the degree of distractedness of the mind. The less distracted it is, the calmer the breathing, while the more distracted, the more restless and irregular the breathing. According to yogic teachings, it is the breath - actually, the movement of the life-force energy or *prana* - that enables the mind to think. If you suspend the breath, the mind loses its fuel and becomes quiet and still. This is what happens in deep meditation, where there is total absorption of the mind.

In the following two sutras, the sage has given us the universal antidote for the obstacles:

> *In order to counteract these distractions, the yogi should practice concentration on a single principle of existence.*
> Yoga Sutras 1:32

The above meditation is not easy, but through perseverance, all ignorance is eliminated. However, a simpler method, for those who find the first antidote difficult, is given:

> *The projection of friendliness, compassion, gladness and*
> *equanimity towards others – whether they bring joy,*
> *sorrow, merit or demerit – will pacify the consciousness.*
> *Yoga Sutras 1:33*

One should always strive to look at all beings with love and compassion, no matter what their relationship or attitude is towards you.

The constant vigilant awareness of the current state of our consciousness will help alert us to the arising of any of the obstacles. The identification of an obstacle is the first step to overcoming it.

Disease

We need a healthy mind in a healthy body so that we can have enough time and opportunity to evolve into the realization of the immortal nature of the Self and fulfill the real purpose of human experience and all the possibilities of life.

Disease arises when there is tension in the body or mind. Disease is the loss of ease, balance and harmony – when the body and mind are in balance, disease cannot occur.

Our spiritual progress can be restricted by a dis-eased mind and body. When you are sick and your body is in pain and feeling weak, it is difficult to sit calmly in meditation. Your mind is distracted by the physical pain and discomfort. You are unable to concentrate or become focused clearly in meditation. This is also due to the mis-identification with the body, for it is not "you" who is sick, but the body. However, in so far, as you identify yourself as the body, then you feel sick.

The mind and body are only instruments of the Self – when they become dis-eased or imbalanced, the Self will not be able to express through them as it would in a healthy mind and physiology.

The mind exerts the deepest influence on the body. With constant awareness and intentional discipline we can consciously create a healthy mind and physiology, maintaining a balance. The following are recommendations for maintaining a natural immunity to disease:

- Exercise regularly – stretch the body, and tone the organs and internal systems
- Breathe properly – learn the full yogic breath, and live away from polluted areas
- Sleep sufficiently such that you get enough rest
- Eat moderately and sufficiently – eat food that is in season and maintain a healthy diet
- Live healthy – drink pure water, breathe pure air
- Maintain a positive outlook on life under all circumstances. Do your best in any circumstance and leave the rest to the Divine.
- Meditate and practice *yama-niyama*

Dullness

This is the consequence of a lack of energy. This energy is an important key to spiritual life. Matter, even our body is only congealed energy. There is a universal store of energy from which we can draw at any time.

Lack of energy can be due to fatigue caused by bad habits, such as working too hard or insufficient sleep. The cultivation of good habits can dramatically increase one's energy level.

A high energy level contributes to a sense of joy. You feel find it difficult to be sad when you are brimming with life and energy. Look at people who are depressed - everyone who is depressed has low energy. One of the most difficult things to do with people who are depressed is to get them to do something about it.

There are also mental blocks which tie up energy and cause a depleted energy level. Unwillingness and fear of failure are all such mental blocks that need to be overcome by will-power and discriminative awareness.

Doubt

Doubt can be positive and expand our awareness, or negative and destructive, resulting in a depressive mood. It depends on your attitude. Healthy doubt leads one to question and dig deeper for profound answers. Unhealthy doubt is that which is unwilling to make the effort to find the answers, or when answers are presented, to accept them after critical examination.

Doubt can lead to a state of confusion, with the mind torn between different and sometimes opposing possibilities.

Doubt can lead to a state of stagnation, without any energy to make a move in any direction.

One must cultivate a healthy sense of doubt, with the willingness to search for and accept reasonable answers. One must also be wise enough to listen to the sages when they all tell us that there are certain questions that cannot be answered by our limited state of consciousness.

Carelessness

We have been brought up with a limited time sense, and encouraged to maximize the productivity of every moment. However, we do this by trying to do multiple things "at the same time" – such as writing and watching television at the same time! Sometimes we try to multiplex ourselves into doing three or even four activities. What an achievement.

Such multiplexing of activities causes carelessness – we cannot put our full attention on any one activity. When such a state of affairs becomes habitual, we become careless in everything we do.

Learn to give your full attention to a single activity, and do it well.

Laziness

This is a state of emotion in which there is a lack of intent to move forward or make progress in any activity. Laziness is caused by inertia which is called *tamas*.

There can be physical laziness and also mental laziness - sometimes the physically lazy person can be excused if the laziness is due to ill health, but mental laziness is inexcusable for those who choose to be unwilling, unmotivated, without self-effort.

To overcome inertia and laziness one needs to purify and "lighten" the physical body and mind to rise to a *sattvic* state. Good habits such as eating healthy vegetarian food, avoiding drugs and exercising regularly helps to "lighten" the physical body. Meditation and breathing techniques can "lighten" the subtle body.

Sensuality

It is necessary to detach from our five senses, the stimuli from the senses and our emotions based on the stimuli. Attachment deepens our desires - attachment to sense-pleasures prevents us from realizing our True Self. Our desire or need for someone or something apart from the Divine creates a sense of separation. If we believe that we can still be satisfied without the presence of the Divine, then our minds are distracted by the 'need' for outer sources of sense stimulation.

Self-control requires first the regulation of our sense-pleasures to bring them into balance, followed by the eventual detachment from them.

False Perception

Ignorance is the cause of false perception. This is the misunderstanding of the impermanent phenomena for the permanent absolute. It is the confusion of the not-self with the True Self, leading to beliefs and actions contrary to that of a sincere spiritual seeker.

The practice of the *niyama* of *svadyaya* or self-study is the best method to overcome the root cause of this false perception. This includes the reading of spiritual classics, listening to the words of sages, and meditating.

Failure to Gain a Firm Ground

This is the failure to progress spiritually due to lack of perseverance, willingness and enthusiasm.

The *siddha* Patanjali has said:

> *Practice becomes firm in ground only when spontaneous awareness continues with consistent efforts without interruption for a long time.*
> Yoga Sutras 1.14

In this culture of fast food and instant gratification, there is a lack of persistence and determination in completing a course of spiritual practice. Very often the seeker flirts with one group and then with another, skimming the practices, without ever penetrating to the depths and drifts away disappointed. Always searching but never satisfied.

This failure to reach a firm ground can only be overcome by the persistent practice of a single course of spiritual teaching to the depth necessary to transform faith into knowing. There is of course a need to use one's power of discrimination at the outset to ensure that the chosen path is credible and trustworthy for the purpose of Self-Realization. The spiritual path is not for those jumping into it with blind faith – such blind faith cannot sustain a prolonged and arduous practice.

Instability

This is caused by the attachment to our emotions. The inability to detach from the emotions causes a life punctuated by the roller-coaster of ups and downs. The alternating current of happiness and grief fries the gate-way to the will-power and discrimination of our innate light, which alone can give calm and happiness.

Instability can only be overcome by the detachment from our emotions. Instead of identifying with our emotions, it is necessary to step aside and be the watcher, to see the motion picture of life for what it is, without getting overly emotional about it.

Self-Discipline

Saucha

Saucha (purity) is the first of the *niyama*. Pure thoughts, positive feelings and the cleanliness of the body are all aspects of *saucha*. While bathing and personal hygiene constitute external cleanliness, the practice of *asanas* (physical postures) and *pranayama* (breath control and expansion) helps us to cleanse our organs of toxins and impurities and our energy and emotional bodies of negativity. With *dhyana* (meditation), the mind is cleansed of impure thoughts.

Yogis and devout people always purify themselves before commencing their prayers and daily activities. Still more important is the cleansing of the *manas* or mind of impure thoughts so that the True Self can shine thought the mirror of the *buddhi*.

One way to think purely is to see the virtues in others and not merely their faults, then the respect which one shows for another's virtues makes one self-respecting as well and helps to overcome personal sorrows and difficulties.

Once there lived a pious and pure man. He lived during the reign of a great king who prided himself on his piety. The king offered fresh flowers and pearls to the Divine in his daily worship. One day while the king was offering his prayers, the pious but extremely poor man arrived at the temple. Unmindful of the king, he sat down to pray. During his worship, the pure man offered to the Lord a few holy basil leaves and some clear, fresh water from an earthen pot.

The proud king was offended when he saw this and berated the poor man, "You poor man, how dare you offer the Lord such

meager offerings? You shall never attain the kingdom of heaven."
"I offer to the Lord all that I have," replied the man meekly.

A little while later, the king was thinking how he could impress his
subjects with his compassion and called his chief minister and asked,
"what acts of giving should I do to please the Lord?" "Why not
make a grand charitable home for the needy and the poor, your
Majesty?" The king was pleased with the suggestion and
commanded work to begin immediately – of course he also asked
his finance minister to levy a tax on the merchants to pay for the
project!

Meanwhile the pious man continued to live an austere life devoted
to prayer and worship. He lived simply and ate only one meal a
day. One day after completing his prayers, the poor man cooked
his food and left it to cool on the window. He then went out for a
short walk. When he returned he found that someone had eaten his
food. The next day the same thing happened. The thefts continued
daily. Deprived of his daily meal the pure man thought, "Perhaps
the Lord wants me to fast."

A few days later, while he was walking around as his food cooled,
he noticed a ragged beggar creeping up to the window. The hungry
wretch stuffed the stolen food into his mouth and then sneaked
away. The pure soul felt very sorry for the starved beggar, and
noticing that the beggar had left the butter uneaten, he ran after
him shouting, "Please wait, you have forgotten to eat the butter!"
But the beggar ran faster, thinking that he was going to get beaten.

Catching up with the beggar, the selfless man pleaded, "Do eat the
butter, too!" The beggar was astonished to see the thin and frail
man parting happily with his food. In an instant, the beggar changed
into his true form. He was none other than the manifested form of
the Lord. "My dear devotee, your purity and selflessness is

unmatched on earth and your suffering on earth is over," said the Lord. The Lord then took him to heaven

A pure mind is always friendly, kind and compassionate, never looking for faults in others but always trying to improve oneself.

One aspect of physical and emotional purity is the food we eat. All living things have a subtle body – a mammal has a more developed subtle body, similar to man, but lacking the fully developed spiritual body while plants only have an energy body and an emotional body. However, everything we eat is not just the physical part that we can see – the meat of a pig or a cow has the subtle body with it even after it has been cooked. The subtle body retains the negative energy and toxic emotions such as fear and anger which accompany the death of the animal. You have to digest the toxic energy and emotions as well as the proteins and other physical constituents. Eating meat is an impure act, not only because it encourages harming of other living beings, but also because of the active ingestion of impure passions!

The spiritual seeker is encouraged to eat less meat, perhaps even becoming a vegetarian. However, lest the vegetarian become too bloated by pride, one must also realize that even plants are living things and feel hurt when plucked and harvested.

Good hygiene and physical cleansing is also an aspect of purity. A long time ago there lived a powerful king in Kashmir. Unfortunately, he was struck down with a disease called leprosy. Physicians and healers were called from far and wide to cure the king, but none of them succeeded.

The king then decided to go on a pilgrimage. He traveled far and wide and met many holy men and saints, but none could help him. At long last he arrived at the temple town of Chidambaram, dedicated to the dancing form of the Lord.

Even though he had been struck down by what was considered an unclean disease, the king still decided to purify himself before entering the shrine and took a dip in the temple tank. When he stepped out of the water, the king noticed that his body had been cleansed of the dreaded disease. His deformities were removed and his whole body sparkled with health and vigor.

The King's joy knew no bounds. Pure in body and mind he offered his thanks to the Lord in the ancient temple. He then made a generous grant whereby the ancient temple was enlarged and made more glorious.

The Practice of Saucha

There are many aspects to attaining purity of the physical, and subtle bodies. We will focus on the primary technique for purifying the subtle energy body.

Pranayama can be used for purifying and removing energy blockages in the subtle body. The main purification breath techniques are called *kabalabathi* and *bhastrika*.

Kapalabhati is 'that which brightens the brain', that is, the brain cells are stimulated by this *pranayama*. We usually inhale actively and exhale passively. This technique reverses the active role, so that exhalation is active and inhalation becomes passive. The focus is on abdominal breathing and the abdominal muscles are used to propel the breath out in a series of fast successive bursts. The posture used can be *vajrasana* [kneeling pose].

Breathe in fully through both nostrils and allow the abdominal muscles to extend slightly. Then pull in the abdominal muscles, and exhale rapidly with a burst of air outward. Allow the abdomen to expand, and let inhalation occur. This is one round.

A minimum of thirty-six rounds should be practiced.

During these exertions, it is still important to keep the spine straight, and not bent in either directions, as muscle spasms in the neck or back may occur, due to the rapid abdominal movements.

The next *pranayama* you should learn is *bhastrika*. The Sanskrit word *bhastrika* means 'bellows'. It's analogous to a blacksmith's bellows which blow air powerfully and rapidly in order to fan the flames of the fire. So to perform this technique, you should inhale and exhale rapidly.

The difference between *bhastrika* and *kapalabhati* is that in *bhastrika*, the inhalation is as rapid as the exhalation, whereas in *kapalabhati*, the inhalation is gentle and long, while the exhalation is rapid and forceful.

Another difference between *bhastrika* and *kapalabhati* is that in *bhastrika,* after inhalation, there is a natural breath retention, until the urge to breathe occurs, during which, there is union of the upward moving life-force *prana* and downward moving life-force *apana.*

Sit comfortably with the spine straight. Relax and close your eyes, keeping a smile on your face.

Inhale and exhale through both nostrils strongly and rapidly, so that the expulsions of breath follow one another in rapid succession. This will bring into rapid action both the diaphragm and the entire respiratory apparatus. One rapid inhalation and exhalation completes one *bhastrika* breath.

Practice sixteen breaths, breathing out deeply on the sixteenth expulsion, and taking a long, slow, deep inhalation through both nostrils.

Then, watch your breath, without forcing the breath retention. Due to the oxygenation of the blood with the rapid breaths, there will be a period during which you will not feel the urge to breathe. Take a normal breath, when the urge arises.

This completes one round of *bhastrika*. Practice a minimum of seven rounds. Take a short rest between each round by taking a few normal breaths. As you progress you can gradually increase the number of breaths from sixteen up to one hundred and forty-four in each round.

People with high blood pressure or heart problems should not practice *bhastrika*.

Santosha

Santosha (Contentment) is the second of the *Niyama*. Contentment and tranquility are states of mind. When the mind cannot become one pointed, it is robbed of its peace. When there is contentment and tranquility the flame of spirit does not waver in the wind of desire. *Santosha* means satisfaction or contentment.

The story of Krishna and his childhood friend Sudama illustrates to us the meaning of contentment. When Krishna was a young boy he studied at the *ashram* or hermitage of Guru Sandipani. Krishna's best friend at the *ashram* was a clever boy named Sudama. The two boys studied, played and grew up together at the *ashram*. On completing their studies the boys were sad to part. After leaving the ashram Krishna had many adventures, and eventually became the king of Dwaraka while Sudama chose to become a priest.

Sudama lived a life of contentment, never desiring for more than he needed. He married a devout lady named Sushila, and in time, his family grew but his earnings as a priest remained small. Sushila found it very difficult to make ends meet. One day there was no food in the house. In despair, Sushila turned to her husband, and said, "our children are hungry and crying. Why don't you go and see your childhood friend, Krishna. He is now a king and will certainly help you."

Sudama just thought that it would be good to see his childhood friend but didn't want to beg money from him. Sushila was very happy that her husband was willing to go for the family. She borrowed some puffed rice from a neighbor and tied it into a cloth bundle, so that he could take a gift for Krishna.

Bearing the humble gift, Sudama set off for distant Dwaraka. After a long walk he arrived at Krishna's capital, and was overwhelmed by the grandeur of the city. He meekly walked up to the palace gates and asked the guard there to tell the king that his friend Sudama had come to visit. The guard couldn't believe that this poor man could be the king's friend, but nevertheless, he conveyed the message to the king.

Krishna was overjoyed to hear that Sudama had come to see him, and rushed to the palace gates, embracing the weary Sudama. Krishna himself washed Sudama's feet and saw to all his comforts. When Krishna noticed the cloth bundle that Sudama had brought with him, he asked him about it. Sudama felt ashamed to offer up his modest present but Krishna grabbed it from him and eagerly opened it. "Puffed rice," he said, "my favorite" and began to eat handfuls of the simple fare.

Sudama was pleased to see that his friend, although now a great king was satisfied with such a humble gift. The two friends talked for hours. At Krishna's request Sudama spent a few days at the palace. Finally remembering that his family would be waiting for him, Sudama took his leave.

He had been so happy to be with his friend, that only while returning in the royal chariot, did Sudama remember the mission for which Sushila had sent him. Both he and Krishna had been so contented with each other's company that neither had brought up his situation or needs. Sudama was now returning empty-handed to his family. Troubled, he got off the chariot a short distance from his hut. As he walked towards his home, he was astounded to find a large mansion where his hut used to stand. Sudama worriedly thought, "Where is my little house and where is my family?" Just then Sushila opened the door, dressed in fine clothes and attended by many servants. She greeted her husband joyously and told him that his friend Krishna had arranged everything while he was away.

Since he no longer had to worry about his family's livelihood, Sudama was content just to live a simple life dedicated to meditation and prayer.

Santosha (contentment) is often described by *yogis* as the "supreme virtue" and as an important practice. Many people, when they hear it described as a virtue at all, are puzzled. To them, contentment seems, if anything, the fruit of virtue rather than a virtue in its own right. If a person lives a good life, it may be assumed that he'll achieve a corresponding measure of contentment.

Those who make this mistake are confusing virtue with passivity. We can become deluded with the false idea that contentment can come only after one has fulfilled every desire. This puts us in a frame of mind where contentment becomes a virtual impossibility! Our constant expectation is of something to be achieved in the future. In this manner we push contentment forever away from us.

Once upon a time, a man gave his son a donkey, but the son was unable to make the stubborn animal move when loaded with goods, no matter how hard he pushed or whipped it. When the son complained to his father, the wise old man tied a carrot on a stick and placed it in front of the dumb donkey, who immediately started to walk quickly, trying to get at the carrot.

Contentment is, in fact, a state of mind. It must be actively practiced, not anticipated for some future time. Our desires are like the carrot before the donkey – when we can see it for what it is, then we can let it go.

It is possible to be contented under all circumstances. Contentment must be a deliberately assumed mental attitude - it doesn't depend on outward circumstances, and in fact the more people anticipate it in the future, the less ability they have to enjoy it fully in the present.

In the history of baseball, it is hard to imagine a greater player with such combination of talent and humility as **Lou Gehrig**. His accomplishments on the field made him an authentic American hero, and his tragic early death made him a legend.

He joined the New York Yankees in 1925, and didn't leave the playing field for over 13 years. Gehrig's consecutive game streak of 2,130 games (a record that stood until Cal Ripken, Jr. broke it in 1995) did not come easily. He played well every day despite a broken thumb, a broken toe and back spasms. Later in his career Gehrig's hands were X-rayed, and doctors were able to spot 17 different fractures that had "healed" while Gehrig continued to play. Despite having pain from lumbago one day, he was listed as the shortstop and leadoff hitter. He singled and was promptly replaced but kept the streak intact. His endurance and strength earned him the nickname "Iron Horse."

Gehrig had spent his whole career in New York, the nation's media capital. But it seemed that another teammate always got more headline attention. First it was Babe Ruth, then later Joe DiMaggio. When historian Fred Lieb asked Gehrig about playing in Ruth's shadow, Gehrig's answer was true to form: "It's a pretty big shadow. It gives me lots of room to spread myself."

Gehrig's play statistics are overwhelming : his lifetime batting average was .340, the 15th all-time highest, and he amassed more than 400 total bases on five occasions. Only 13 men have achieved that level of power in a season. Ruth did it twice, and Chuck Klein did it three times. Gehrig is one of only seven players with more than 100 extra-base hits in one season, and only he and Klein accomplished that feat twice.

During his career, Gehrig averaged 147 RBIs a season. No other player was to reach the 147 mark in a single season until George Foster did it in 1977. And, as historian Bill Curran points out, Gehrig accomplished it "while batting immediately behind two of history's greatest base-cleaners, Ruth and DiMaggio." Gehrig's 184 RBIs in 1931 remains the highest single season total in American League history.

Gehrig won the Triple Crown in 1934, with a .363 average, 49 homers and 165 RBI and was chosen Most Valuable Player again in 1936. He batted .361 in 34 World Series games with 10 homers, eight doubles and 35 RBIs. He also holds the record for career grand slams at 23. He hit 73 three-run homers and 166 two-run shots, giving him the highest average of RBI per homer of any player with more than 300 home runs.

In 1939, when he was only 36 years old, doctors at the Mayo Clinic diagnosed Gehrig with a very rare form of degenerative disease: amyotrophic lateral sclerosis (ALS), which is now called Lou Gehrig's disease. There was no chance he would ever play baseball again. New York sportswriter Paul Gallico suggested the team have a recognition day to honor Gehrig on July 4, 1939. There were more than 62,000 fans in attendance as Gehrig stood on the field at Yankee Stadium with the 1927 and 1939 Yankees. His farewell speech showed his humility and deep contentment, even in the face of life dealing such a blow when he was still in his prime:

> *Fans, for the past two weeks you have been reading about the bad break I got. Yet today I consider myself the luckiest man on the face of this earth. I have been in ballparks for seventeen years and have never received anything but kindness and encouragement from you fans.*

> *"Look at these grand men. Which of you wouldn't consider it the highlight of his career just to associate with them for even one day? Sure, I'm lucky. Who wouldn't consider it an honor to have known Jacob Ruppert? Also, the builder of baseball's greatest empire, Ed Barrow? To have spent six years with that wonderful little fellow, Miller Huggins? Then to have spent the next nine years with that outstanding leader, that smart student of psychology, the best manager in baseball today, Joe McCarthy? Sure, I'm lucky.*

"When the New York Giants, a team you would give your right arm to beat, and vice versa, sends you a gift - that's something. When everybody down to the groundskeepers and those boys in white coats remember you with trophies - that's something. When you have a wonderful mother-in-law who takes sides with you in squabbles with her own daughter - that's something. When you have a father and a mother who work all their lives so you can have an education and build your body - it's a blessing. When you have a wife who has been a tower of strength and shown more courage than you dreamed existed - that's the finest I know.

"So I close in saying that I may have had a tough break, but I have an awful lot to live for."

The practice of Santosha

Contentment is an active state which can be cultivated by practicing mindfulness and constant self-awareness in order to stay in the present – the here and now.

Without attentive awareness and alertness, our consciousness becomes clouded, we become sleepy and our senses lose their sensitivity and become dull. When our attention and sensitivity are sharpened and heightened with awareness, our perception becomes clear. In this state of observation we are able to perceive and recognize those limiting conditions and can understand why the mind is distracted and inattentive. In unbroken, clear awareness we can de-condition and de-hypnotize the mind of its subconscious grasping after some future gratification of desires.

Self-awareness begins with you here and now in this moment, in every moment of your life. When you live every moment in awareness, you will experience the Eternal as a living reality. The average person only uses a tiny fraction of awareness in his or her everyday living. We go from one day to the next throughout life in a state of distraction, unawareness and restlessness. We are sleeping with our eyes open, unaware of the beauty around us.

In the conditioned state of mind we are subject to our subconscious motives, and therefore our perceptions are distorted. We are not even aware or mindful when eating our meals or listening when someone is talking to us. How often do people leave water running from a tap, or forget to switch a light or heater off before going out. These may seem like inconsequential small activities in one's life, but the way to self-realization requires the sensitivity, awareness, care and attention to all that we do in thought, word and action - no matter how small it may seem. We need to live each moment of our life completely, carefully observing all the details with constant awareness and attention.

The sages constantly remind us that it does not matter how long you have been sitting in the dark ... when light is brought in, the darkness disappears. It is our responsibility to awake in the light, to consciously know our true nature and reality as the Self. It is through mastery of our mind, body and senses, that we can direct our lives intelligently and super-consciously, expressing our selves in a balanced and fulfilling way on all levels of our being.

Self-knowledge is the awareness of the immortal reality within us, which sets us free from the bondage of ignorance, the cause of all our sorrows. This knowledge and awareness, which is the Self, is here and now, always. It has never ceased to be, and so is not a goal that we have to search for.

There is no mystery to it. All we need to do is remove the obstacles, dispelling the ignorance that obscures the Self as knowledge. The sun is always shining, but when it is obscured by dark clouds we do not see it. When the clouds disperse then the sun becomes visible and the light shines.

The past is gone and cannot be changed, while the future is not yet and cannot be known – all we have is the present. Yet we brood about the past and fear for the future, forgetting to live in the present. Let us resolve to be mindful and live life in the Here and Now.

Tapas

Tapas is the third *niyama*. *Tapas* means penance, austerity or a burning effort. *Tapas* is derived from the root 'tap' meaning to blaze, burn, shine, suffer pain or consume by heat. It therefore means a burning effort under all circumstances to achieve a definite goal in life. It is transformation which involves purification, self discipline and austerity. The whole science of Yoga may be regarded as a practice of *tapas*. In point of fact, even the path of Self-Realization is in essence the practice of *tapas*.

It is not unusual for great sages and yogis to be renowned for their *tapas*, but there is a boy named Dhruva who is still remembered for the difficult penance he practiced. Dhruva's father was a great king who had two wives. The elder queen was called Suniti – a modest and kind lady who was Dhruva's mother. The second wife, Surichi was ambitious and wished to ensure that her son would be the king's successor. She therefore took every opportunity to belittle the elder queen and her innocent son Dhruva. The king believed Surichi's tales and showered all his affections on the younger queen and her son.

One day finding his father alone, Dhruva went and sat on his lap. When Surichi came and saw this, she was outraged and pulled Dhruva out of his father's lap, screaming that he was not worthy to sit on the king's lap. Dhruva was hurt and went crying to his mother, vowing that he would practice austerities until he attained a position higher even than that of his father!

Despite the pleas of his mother, the strong willed boy held steadfastly to his promise. Finally Dhruva obtained his mother's blessings and left for the forest. Although he was only a boy, Dhruva wandered alone in the forest in search of a teacher. Whenever Dhruva met wise and holy men he would ask them to show him the path to heaven. Some wisemen admired his courage, others laughed at him and still others asked him to return home. None, however would show him the path sought, since he was considered too young.

The unwavering Dhruva continued his search. He lived on wild fruits, berries and water. Neither heat nor cold, neither wild beasts nor hunger could deter him from his efforts. Then one day Dhruva met the wise sage, Narada, who taught him a prayer:

"If you wish to reach heaven," said Narada, "chant this prayer and meditate on the Lord."

Dhruva was happy for the guidance. He sat cross-legged under a tree and concentrated his thoughts and feelings on the Lord. For days on end he meditated, prayed and fasted. Finally, greatly moved by the child's burning efforts and austerities, the Lord appeared before him.

"O Lord," the boy prayed, "Please remove all of my mother's sorrows and grant me a place in heaven."

"Dhruva," said Lord, "your practice has been more severe than that of great sages. I shall grant you your wish. Now return home to your mother."

Young Dhruva returned home with a large following. His parents were delighted to see him. Surichi apologized for having mistreated him. When Dhruva came of age, his father crowned him as a king. Dhruva wisely governed his kingdom for many years. When he grew old the Lord raised him to the heaven and made him a bright star called Dhruva - the Pole Star.

Practice of Tapas

> *"Unearned suffering is redemptive.*
> *Suffering, the nonviolent resister realizes,*
> *has tremendous educational and transforming possibilities."*
> Martin Luther King, Jr.

Physical austerity: Fasting is highly recommended as a means to control the body. We eat sometimes out of habit and sometimes from desire. There is great resistance against skipping even one meal, not to mention going without food for a day or two. In ancient times, fasting was regularly practiced as a means to cleanse the body of toxins, as well as to develop self-control. Start with eating one less meal during the day; then try taking only liquids for a whole day; progress to one whole day (preferably a day when you are not working, such as a Saturday or Sunday) without food. Drink plenty of water during the fast, and be mindful of your thoughts and emotions.

Mental austerity: *Mauna* – the practice of Silence takes great discipline and can build up a lot of spiritual fire. Many sages have practiced silence, sometimes for years or even a life-time, and are called *munis*. It has been shown that such practice can develop profound changes in consciousness. Start off by practicing silence for half a day and progress to a whole day or even a whole week. It becomes easier with time, as the outer silence can lead to inner silence and even to a center of bliss – you might even be reluctant to begin talking again after the experience. Practice this regularly, at least once a month.

Bhuta Shuddhi – **purification of the Elements of the body:**

Since both the physical and subtle bodies are composed of combinations of the principle of consciousness with the five cosmic elements of space, air, fire, water and earth, a purification of these elements is beneficial.

This *pranayama* utilizes a ratio of [16:0:32:0], that is the exhalation is twice as long as the inhalation which should have a duration of sixteen counts and there is no holding of breath in between. The *chakra bija mantras* or sound formulae for the cosmic elements of air, fire, consciousness, and earth are silently repeated with the breath.

Sit in any firm posture with the back straight, and utilize the fingers of the right hand to for alternating the left and right nostrils.

Be aware of your heart center, and inhale through the left nostril and mentally repeat *yam*, the *bija* or seed *mantra* of the element of Air, for a count of sixteen seconds.

Watch your breath, and mentally repeat the *mantra yam*, until you have the urge to breathe. Do not try to hold your breath. Then, exhale through the right nostril, mentally repeating *yam* thirty-two times.

Watch your breath, and mentally repeat the *mantra yam*, until you have the urge to breathe.

Now move your awareness to the navel center. Inhale through your right nostril, mentally repeating *ram*, the *bija mantra* of Fire sixteen times with the breath.

Watch your breath, and mentally repeat the *mantra ram*, until you have the urge to breathe. Then, exhale through the left nostril, mentally repeating *ram* thirty-two times.

Watch your breath, and mentally repeat the *mantra ram*, until you have the urge to breathe.

Move your awareness to the third-eye center, inside your head, behind the point between the eyebrows. Inhale through your left nostril, mentally repeating *om*, the *bija mantra* of Consciousness, sixteen times, with the breath.

Watch your breath, and mentally repeat the *mantra om*, until you have the urge to breathe. Then, exhale through the left nostril, mentally repeating *om* thirty-two times. Watch your breath, and mentally repeat the *mantra om*, until you have the urge to breathe.

Move your awareness to the root center. Inhale through the right nostril, mentally repeating *lam*, the *bija mantra* of Earth sixteen times. Repeat the *mantra lam* until you need to breathe, and then exhale through the left nostril, mentally repeating *lam* thirty-two times.

This completes one round. Practice a minimum of 3 rounds.

Svadhyaya

Svadhyaya is the fourth *niyama* - it means Self-Study or to know one's self. *Svadhyaya* is not just attending a lecture where the lecturer parades his own learning and gives instructions or doctrines to his audience. When people meet for *svadhyaya*, the speaker and listener are of one mind and have mutual love and respect.

As the aspirant becomes more and more established in the first three *niyamas* – *saucha, santosha* and *tapas* – there is a gradual deepening into self-study with awareness. In self-study one learns not by gaining intellectual or material knowledge but by standing aside to observe, and to study the studier. It is by observing with awareness one's own thoughts, feelings, behavior, desires and motives. It is by observing that attitudes that prevent us from realizing our true Self. The practice of svadhaya enables spiritual awakening in us, so that we can realize our divine nature.

At the deepest level of our inner Being we are pure consciousness, a spark of the Divine. If we do not know this, it is because of self-forgetfulness and ignorance due to identification with the mind and the objects of the senses. All our problems in life ultimately stem from our separation from the Divine Source.

Most people live an outward life - primarily for themselves and their families – this is the conditioning from our parents and role models or authority figures in society teaching us to look outside of ourselves for happiness and fulfillment. But the great Masters have given us a different message:

> *Jesus said: "The Kingdom of God is within you."*
> Matthew 6:33

Lord Krishna said: To those who meditate on Me as their very own, ever united to Me by incessant worship, I provide for their deficiencies and make permanent their gain.
Bhagavat Gita 9:22

The Divine which is Truth, Consciousness and Bliss is within each one of us. Each one of us is an expression of Divine Consciousness, but until we awaken to this essential fact and experience the reality of our true nature, we cannot express the Divine within us.

Svadhaya also means the study of scriptural texts and the silent recitation of *mantras* to oneself. The mental repetition of mantras in this way is called *japa*. Both the study of scriptural texts and *mantra japa* are to be practiced in a meditative and concentrated state of absorbed awareness

To make life healthy, happy and calm, it is essential to regularly study inspirational literature in a peaceful place. This will help an aspirant to concentrate upon and solve the difficult problems of life when they arise. Such a study is a means to put an end to ignorance and bring knowledge. Ignorance has no beginning, but can have an end. It is recommended to follow the example of the honey-bee who savors the nectar in various flowers – in the same way an aspiring *yogi* absorbs the truths in all faiths enabling the transcendence of all religions.

There is a story of another young boy named Nachiketa who provides a good example of somebody who really wanted to know and understand himself. Nachiketa's father was sage Vajashravasa, once conducted a great ceremony, in which he offered all he had. He had used all he owned to buy cows, but because of his poverty, he could only afford lean and old cows. In order to honor his father, the boy bravely offered himself as part of the offering.

The little boy asked, "Father, who will you give me to?" At first his father would not reply, but Nachiketa persisted with the question. Since the old man had recently been pondering on the mysteries of death, he muttered angrily, "I give you to the god of death." Undaunted, Nachiketa marched off and after much effort and hardship, found the palace of Yama, the God of death.

Yama, who is also called Dharmaraja or lord of the law, was away and so Nachiketa waited, fasting and praying. Three days later when Yama returned to find a fearless boy standing at his palace gates, Death was pleased with the lad's devotion and determination.

"Since you have waited for three days I shall grant you three boons," he told Nachiketa.

"First, let my father be happy when I return to him on earth," requested Nachiketa. "Granted," answered Yama. "Next tell me how to get to heaven?" asked Nachiketa. Yama then taught Nachiketa how to attain the sorrow-less world called heaven.

Finally, the boy asked Death to explain what happens to a man after he dies, because he wanted to attain to the deathless state. Yama, was taken aback, and reluctant to reveal such secrets to a mortal. "Ask for anything else, herds of cattle, many elephants, gold, palaces and a long life." He urged.

"Oh no, I don't want any of these things!" Nachiketa persisted. "Tell me - does a man continue to exist after he dies?"

Finally, after his best efforts to change the boy's mind had failed, Yama was convinced of Nachiketa's keen desire to understand the mysteries of life and death, and assented to instruct him further.

"The soul continues to exist though the body dies and decays, explained Yama, "it is like a rider and your body is like a chariot.

Your intelligence is the charioteer and your thoughts and feelings are the reins. Your five senses - sight, hearing, smell, taste and touch are the five horses that draw the chariot. The world around you is like the pastures on which these horses graze."

Then Yama taught Nachiketa the importance of Yoga. He explained how by practicing Yoga, the aspirant can bring his senses under control just as a charioteer brings his horses under control. As soon as one has controlled the senses, one will see the soul and experience the true Self. Nachiketa was the best disciple Death ever had and learnt well what Yama taught him. He made a deep effort to achieve his true nature and achieved Self-Realization, becoming a perfected being.

The Practice of Svadhaya

The following is the essence of self-enquiry as taught by the sage of Arunachala, Ramana Maharshi:

All living beings desire to be always happy, without misery. In the case of everyone there is observed a supreme love for one's Self – truly happiness is the cause for love. Therefore, to gain that happiness which is one's nature and which is experienced in the state of deep sleep where there is no mind, one should know one's Self. For that, the path of knowledge, the inquiry of the form "Who am I?" is the principal means.

1. Who am I?

The gross body which is composed of the seven humors (dhatus), I am not; the five cognitive sense organs, namely the senses of hearing, touch, sight, taste, and smell, which apprehend their respective objects, viz. sound, touch, color, taste, and odor, I am not; the five cognitive sense-organs, namely the organs of speech, locomotion, grasping, excretion, and procreation, which have as their respective functions speaking, moving, grasping, excreting, and enjoying, I am not; the five vital airs, prana, etc., which perform respectively the five functions of in-breathing, etc., I am not; even the mind which thinks, I am not; the nescience too, which is endowed only with the residual impressions of objects, and in which there are no objects and no functioning's, I am not.

2. If I am none of these, then who am I?

After the negation of all of the above mentioned as 'not this', 'not this', that Awareness which alone remains - that I am.

3. What is the nature of Awareness?

The nature of Awareness is Existence-Consciousness-Bliss

4. When will the realization of the Self be gained?

When the world which is what-is-seen has been removed, there will be realization of the Self which is the seer.

5. Will there not be realization of the Self even while the world is there (taken as real)?

There will not be.

6. Why?

The seer and the object seen are like the rope and the snake. Just as the knowledge of the rope which is the substrate will not arise unless the false knowledge of the illusory serpent goes, so the realization of the Self which is the substrate will not be gained unless the belief that the world is real is removed.

7. When will the world which is the object seen be removed?

When the mind, which is the cause of all cognition's and of all actions, becomes quiescent, the world will disappear.

8. What is the nature of the mind?

What is called 'mind' is a wondrous power residing in the Self. It causes all thoughts to arise. Apart from thoughts, there is no such thing as mind. Therefore, thought is the nature of mind. Apart from thoughts, there is no independent entity called the world. In deep sleep there are no thoughts, and there is no world. In the states of waking and dream, there are thoughts, and there is a world also. Just as the spider emits the thread (of the web) out of itself and again withdraws it into itself, likewise the mind projects the world out of itself and again resolves it into itself. When the mind comes out of the Self, the world appears. Therefore, when the world appears (to be real), the Self does not appear; and when the Self appears (shines) the world does not appear. When one persistently inquires into the nature of the mind, the mind will end leaving the Self (as the residue). What is referred to as the Self is the Atman. The mind always exists only in dependence on something gross; it cannot stay alone. It is the mind that is called the subtle body or the soul (jiva).

9. What is the path of inquiry for understanding the nature of the mind?

That which rises as 'I' in this body is the mind. If one inquires as to where in the body the thought 'I' rises first, one would discover that it rises in the heart. That is the place of the mind's origin. Even if one thinks constantly 'I' 'I', one will be led to that place. Of all the thoughts that arise in the mind, the 'I' thought is the first. It is only after the rise of this that the other thoughts arise. It is after the appearance of the first personal pronoun that the second and third personal pronouns appear; without the first personal pronoun there will not be the second and third.

10. How will the mind become quiescent?

By the inquiry 'Who am I?'. The thought 'who am I?' will destroy all other thoughts, and like the stick used for stirring the burning pyre, it will itself in the end get destroyed. Then, there will arise Self-realization.

11. What is the means for constantly holding on to the thought 'Who am I?'

When other thoughts arise, one should not pursue them, but should inquire: 'To whom do they arise?' It does not matter how many thoughts arise. As each thought arises, one should inquire with diligence, 'To whom has this thought arisen?". The answer that would emerge would be "To me". Thereupon if one inquires "Who am I?", the mind will go back to its source; and the thought that arose will become quiescent. With repeated practice in this manner, the mind will develop the skill to stay in its source. When the mind that is subtle goes out through the brain and the sense-organs, the gross names and forms appear; when it stays in the heart, the names and forms disappear. Not letting the mind go out, but retaining it in the Heart is what is called "inwardness" (antar-mukha). Letting the mind go out of the Heart is known as "externalization" (bahir-mukha). Thus, when the mind stays in the Heart, the 'I' which is the source of all thoughts will go, and the Self which ever exists will shine. Whatever one does, one should do without the egoity "I". If one acts in that way, all will appear as of the nature of Shiva (God).

12. Are there no other means for making the mind quiescent?

Other than inquiry, there are no adequate means. If through other means it is sought to control the mind, the mind will appear to be controlled, but will again go forth. Through the control of breath also, the mind will become quiescent; but it will be quiescent only so long as the breath remains controlled, and when the breath resumes the mind also will again start moving and will wander as impelled by residual impressions. The source is the same for both mind and breath. Thought, indeed, is the nature of the mind. The thought 'I' is the first thought of the mind; and that is egoity. It is from that whence egoity originates that breath also originates. Therefore, when the mind becomes quiescent, the breath is controlled, and when the breath is controlled the mind becomes quiescent. But in deep sleep, although the mind becomes quiescent, the breath does not stop. This is because of the will of God, so that the body may be preserved and other people may not be under the impression that it is dead. In the state of waking and in samadhi, when the mind becomes quiescent the breath is controlled. Breath is the gross form of mind. Till the time of death, the mind keeps breath in the body; and when the body dies the mind takes the breath along with it. Therefore, the exercise of breath-control is only an aid for rendering the mind quiescent (manonigraha); it will not destroy the mind (manonasa).

Like the practice of breath-control. meditation on the forms of God, repetition of mantras, restriction on food, etc., are but aids for rendering the mind quiescent.

Through meditation on the forms of God and through repetition of mantras, the mind becomes one-pointed. The mind will always be wandering. Just as when a chain is given to an elephant to hold in its trunk it will go along grasping the chain and nothing else, so also when the mind is occupied with a name or form it will grasp that alone. When the mind expands in the form of countless thoughts, each thought becomes weak; but as thoughts get resolved the mind becomes one-pointed and strong; for such a mind Self-inquiry will become easy. Of all the restrictive rules, that relating to the taking of sattvic food in moderate quantities is the best; by observing this rule, the sattvic quality of mind will increase, and that will be helpful to Self-inquiry.

13. The residual impressions (thoughts) of objects appear wending like the waves of an ocean. When will all of them get destroyed?

As the meditation on the Self rises higher and higher, the thoughts will get destroyed.

14. Is it possible for the residual impressions of objects that come from beginning-less time, as it were, to be resolved, and for one to remain as the pure Self?

Without yielding to the doubt "Is it possible, or not?", one should persistently hold on to the meditation on the Self. Even if one be a great sinner, one should not worry and weep "O! I am a sinner, how can I be saved?"; one should completely renounce the thought "I am a sinner"; and concentrate keenly on meditation on the Self; then, one would surely succeed. There are not two minds - one good and the other evil; the mind is only one. It is the residual impressions that are of two kinds - auspicious and inauspicious. When the mind is under the influence of auspicious impressions it is called good; and when it is under the influence of inauspicious impressions it is regarded as evil.

The mind should not be allowed to wander towards worldly objects and what concerns other people. However bad other people may be, one should bear no hatred for them. Both desire and hatred should be eschewed. All that one gives to others one gives to one's self. If this truth is understood who will not give to others? When one's self arises all arises; when one's self becomes quiescent all becomes quiescent. To the extent we behave with humility, to that extent there will result good. If the mind is rendered quiescent, one may live anywhere.

15. How long should inquiry be practiced?

As long as there are impressions of objects in the mind, so long the inquiry "Who am I?" is required. As thoughts arise they should be destroyed then and there in the very place of their origin, through inquiry. If one resorts to contemplation of the Self non-intermittently, until the Self is gained, that alone would do. As long as there are enemies within the fortress, they will continue to sally forth; if they are destroyed as they emerge, the fortress will fall into our hands.

16. What is the nature of the Self?

What exists in truth is the Self alone. The world, the individual soul, and God are appearances in it, like silver in mother-of-pearl, these three appear at the same time, and disappear at the same time. The Self is that where there is absolutely no "I" thought. That is called "Silence". The Self itself is the world; the Self itself is "I"; the Self itself is God; all is Shiva, the Self.

17. Is not everything the work of God?

Without desire, resolve, or effort, the sun rises; and in its mere presence, the sun-stone emits fire, the lotus blooms, water evaporates; people perform their various functions and then rest. Just as in the presence of the magnet the needle moves, it is by virtue of the mere presence of God that the souls governed by the three (cosmic) functions or the fivefold divine activity perform their actions and then rest, in accordance with their respective karmas. God has no resolve; no karma attaches itself to Him. That is like worldly actions not affecting the sun, or like the merits and demerits of the other four elements not affecting all pervading space.

18. Of the devotees, who is the greatest?

He who gives himself up to the Self that is God is the most excellent devotee. Giving one's self up to God means remaining constantly in the Self without giving room for the rise of any thoughts other than that of the Self. Whatever burdens are thrown on God, He bears them. Since the supreme power of God makes all things move, why should we, without submitting ourselves to it, constantly worry ourselves with thoughts as to what should be done and how, and what should not be done and how not? We know that the train carries all loads, so after getting on it why should we carry our small luggage on our head to our discomfort, instead of putting it down in the train and feeling at ease?

19. What is non-attachment?

As thoughts arise, destroying them utterly without any residue in the very place of their origin is non-attachment. Just as the pearl-diver ties a stone to his waist, sinks to the bottom of the sea and there takes the pearls, so each one of us should be endowed with non-attachment, dive within oneself and obtain the Self-Pearl.

20. Is it not possible for God and the Guru to effect the release of a soul?

God and the Guru will only show the way to release; they will not by themselves take the soul to the state of release. In truth, God and the Guru are not different. Just as the prey which has fallen into the jaws of a tiger has no escape, so those who have come within the ambit of the Guru's gracious look will be saved by the Guru and will not get lost; yet, each one should by his own effort pursue the path shown by God or Guru and gain release. One can know oneself only with one's own eye of knowledge, and not with somebody else's. Does he who is Rama require the help of a mirror to know that he is Rama?

21. Is it necessary for one who longs for release to inquire into the nature of categories (*tattvas*)?

Just as one who wants to throw away garbage has no need to analyze it and see what it is, so one who wants to know the Self has no need to count the number of categories or inquire into their characteristics; what he has to do is to reject altogether the categories that hide the Self. The world should be considered like a dream.

22. Is there no difference between waking and dream?

Waking is long and a dream short; other than this there is no difference. Just as waking happenings seem real while awake, so do those in a dream while dreaming. In dream the mind takes on another body. In both waking and dream states thoughts, names and forms occur simultaneously.

23. Is it any use reading books for those who long for release?

All the texts say that in order to gain release one should render the mind quiescent; therefore their conclusive teaching is that the mind should be rendered quiescent; once this has been understood there is no need for endless reading. In order to quieten the mind one has only to inquire within oneself what one's Self is; how could this search be done in books? One should know one's Self with one's own eye of wisdom. The Self is within the five sheaths; but books are outside them. Since the Self has to be inquired into by discarding the five sheaths, it is futile to search for it in books. There will come a time when one will have to forget all that one has learned.

24. What is happiness?

Happiness is the very nature of the Self; happiness and the Self are not different. There is no happiness in any object of the world.

We imagine through our ignorance that we derive happiness from objects. When the mind goes out, it experiences misery. In truth, when its desires are fulfilled, it returns to its own place and enjoys the happiness that is the Self. Similarly, in the states of sleep, samadhi and fainting, and when the object desired is obtained or the object disliked is removed, the mind becomes inward-turned, and enjoys pure Self-Happiness. Thus the mind moves without rest alternately going out of the Self and returning to it. Under the tree the shade is pleasant; out in the open the heat is scorching. A person who has been going about in the sun feels cool when he reaches the shade. Someone who keeps on going from the shade into the sun and then back into the shade is a fool. A wise man stays permanently in the shade. Similarly, the mind of the one who knows the truth does not leave Brahman. The mind of the ignorant, on the contrary, revolves in the world, feeling miserable, and for a little time returns to Brahman to experience happiness. In fact, what is called the world is only thought. When the world disappears, i.e. when there is no thought, the mind experiences happiness; and when the world appears, it goes through misery.

25. What is wisdom-insight (*jnana-drsti*)?

Remaining quiet is what is called wisdom-insight. To remain quiet is to resolve the mind in the Self. Telepathy, knowing past, present and future happenings and clairvoyance do not constitute wisdom-insight.

26. What is the relation between desirelessness and wisdom?

Desirelessness is wisdom. The two are not different; they are the same. Desirelessness is refraining from turning the mind towards any object. Wisdom means the appearance of no object. In other words, not seeking what is other than the Self is detachment or desirelessness; not leaving the Self is wisdom.

27. What is the difference between inquiry and meditation?

Inquiry consists in retaining the mind in the Self. Meditation consists in thinking that one's self is Brahman, existence-consciousness-bliss.

28. What is release?

Inquiring into the nature of one's self that is in bondage, and realizing one's true nature is release.

When you awaken to your nature within, you will grow into the light, which will remove all darkness and unknowing from the mind and consciousness. With soul-awareness immersed in the Divine you will be able to control your own destiny, living a life guided by the divine spirit within, governed by truth.

Patanjali, in his Yoga Sutras instructs us how to remove ignorance effectively: 'the practice of uninterrupted awareness and discrimination between what is real and what is unreal, removes obstacles [ignorance],' (2:26).

The Divine cannot be completely understood or realized through the intellectual process. Self-study must begin with awareness and an understanding of the mind's movements, the study of the nature of thought and the thinking process. What is thought? How does it arise? What are its functions and limitations? Self-study is not an intellectual process, but simply a perceptive awareness of the movements of the mind, which arises through our distraction from moment to moment. When we recognize our distraction or lack of awareness we can discover our true identity and reality as it is. All that is needed is simple attention to what is happening in us and around us in each moment. Whether we are breathing, meditating, chanting, cooking, eating, working or studying, if we do it with attentive awareness and alertness, each moment will be a freeing experience, in which we will see and understand something new.

Life requires of us to be constantly in clear awareness; with a quiet, meditative mind, which is full of energy, love and compassion, a mind that is free from past conditioning, reactive behavior, sense-urges negative emotions and negative attitudes. In the quiet, aware and alert mind there is true freedom from tension, conflict and sorrow. There is a direct perception of life without distortion.

The intelligent practice of the first seven of the eight limbs of yoga with uninterrupted awareness, gives us the basic methods in removing ignorance. If we are to remain in the light of Self-knowledge, then we need to be vigilant, constantly awake, alert and aware in every moment. This is no part-time exercise: the practice of Yoga once taken up, involves your entire life. If we are unmotivated, uncommitted and practicing only half-heartedly we cannot expect complete success and fulfillment in this incarnation. A total approach to the spiritual life with complete commitment to awakening in Divine Consciousness is required for awakening from ignorance of the True Self.

Ishvara Pranidhana

Ishvara Pranidhana (dedication to the Lord of one's actions and one's will) is the fifth and last *niyama*. *Ishvara Pranidhana* means faith in the Divine. He who has faith in the Divine does not despair. He has illumination. He who knows that all creation belongs to the Lord will not be puffed up with pride or drunk with power. He will not stop for selfish purposes, his head will bow only in worship. Addiction to pleasures destroys both power and glory. When the mind has been emptied of desires of personal gratification, it should be filled with thoughts of the Lord. In a mind filled with thoughts of personal gratification, the senses drag the mind after the objects of desire. Attempts to practice surrender to the Divine without emptying the mind of desire is like building a fire with wet wood.

There is an amazing story of a boy named Prahlada, the same who when grown up challenged the god Indra for Lordship of the three worlds in the story earlier in the book. This Prahlada, though born of demon parents, had tremendous faith in the Divine. King Hiranya-Kashyapu, who controlled a vast empire was a powerful demon. He hated Lord Vishnu because Vishnu had killed his twin brother. One day he summoned his ministers and said, "destroy all temples and images of Vishnu in my kingdom. Burn all books bearing Vishnu's name and make sure that no one chants his name in my domain."

The King wished to ensure that his little boy, Prahlada would grow up to be a fierce demon. Therefore he entrusted Prahlada to a renowned teacher saying, "Initiate the boy into all the demonic ways, teach him to despise the gods and make sure he never hears the name of Vishnu."

Several months later, desiring to know how his son was doing in his studies, the king sent for Prahlada, "Boy, what have you learned so far?" "I have learned to adore the name of Vishnu," said the innocent child. "What!" cried his father the King, hardly able to believe his ears. He called for the boy's teacher and ordered that his head be chopped off for disobedience.

Groveling in fear, the teacher protested his innocence, crying out, "Pardon me my Lord, I did not teach Prahlada to adore Vishnu." "If your teacher didn't, then who taught you that dreadful name?" thundered the King.

"Lord Vishnu himself taught me," replied the devout Prahlada. "Take this boy away," fumed the King, "and rid him of this nonsense which he has learned." Disillusioned the King left Prahlada to his studies for a few more years.

The tyrant once again summoned the boy and questioned him, "Now have you learned anything sensible?" "I bow to the great Lord Vishnu," the pious boy said to his father. The furious King could not contain himself and ordered his demon soldiers to kill the boy. The soldiers attacked Prahlada with sharp-edged swords and heavy clubs, but the calm boy stood calmly chanting the name of Lord Vishnu, and with the Lord's protection remained uninjured by the blows. The enraged King then ordered his soldiers to throw his son into a pit full of poisonous snakes. Prahlada stood fearlessly amidst the serpents and still chanting Lord Vishnu's name remained unharmed.

Finally, the demon king ordered that the boy be thrown into the fire – but of course the devout Prahlada came out of the fire unharmed. The tyrant had no choice but to let his son go on his way.

On another day as the faithful boy was chanting his prayers, the demon king was moved to challenge him, "You silly boy, since you say Vishnu is everywhere, show him to me in this pillar!"

This was just what the Lord was waiting for, and with a terrible roar burst out of the pillar in the form of half man and half lion –

the *avatar* Nirsimha. He killed the tyrannical king and blessed his little devotee. The pious Prahlada was then crowned King.

Practice of Surrender to the Divine: *Bhakti*

This is the practice as well as the state of spiritual devotion to the Divine. It is not an ephemeral emotional state, but a constant turning of one's energies towards the Divine.

According to the *Bhakti Sutras*, a pre-eminent text on this practice:

> *Spiritual devotion is developed by relinquishing objects and relinquishing attachments.*
> Bhakti Sutras 35

There is no room for attachments to any objects or desires – there is only the fullness of Divine in one's life. For there to be devotion to the Lord, one must develop the purity of the *yamas,* leading to contentment and equanimity.

Accordingly, in *sutra* 7, 8,9,10, it is stated:

> *Spiritual devotion does not arise from desire. Its nature is a state of inner stillness.*

> *This inner stillness consecrates the performance of worldly and traditional social duties.*

> *Inner stillness furthermore requires a single-hearted intention and disinterest in what is antagonistic to spiritual devotion.*

> *When one is single-hearted, one relinquishes seeking security in anything other than the Divine.*

There is a story about the Lord of Yoga, Shiva, coming down from the lofty heights in the Himalayas, together with his partner Parvati, to visit with the student *yogis*. The Lord was there to check on their spiritual progress, to give helpful pointers and encouragement to those striving for Self-Realization.

At one hermitage, there were a number of very advanced *yogis* who practiced day and night. One old servant dutifully took care of their needs. Since the old servant was not able to practice any advanced techniques, all he did was to repeat the name of the Lord – 'Namashivaya', and he was content.

While Lord Shiva was visiting them, each *yogi* came to him and asked him about their progress and how much longer they must practice before enlightenment. To all of them He would praise them for their efforts, and to one, he would say, three more lives, to a second, two more lives and to a third, one more life… however, all the yogis felt unhappy and wished that they could achieve liberation in that life-time. However, they kept quiet.

At last when the Lord was leaving, the old servant humbly approached Him and also asked about his own progress. The Lord saw that it would take another thousand lives before the old man would achieve Self-Realization, but did not want to discourage him, and only said, "My son, you are making good progress, and sooner or later, you will be with me."

The old man then began to dance about, repeating the Lord's name and giving thanks. No sooner did he did he do this, that the old man suddenly become young and was transported to the abode of the Lord in a blaze of light.

Parvati was puzzled and asked Lord Shiva what had happened. The Lord then responded that the old man had given up all attachments, even that for liberation, and was totally single-hearted in seeking security in the Divine, and by trusting totally in His words, was instantly transformed.

Such is the power of non-attachment and single-hearted devotion. As far as some actions that can be done to develop devotion, it is stated:

> *By unceasing worship; as well as singing and listening to*
> *the attributes of the Divine.*
> *Bhakti Sutras 36,37*

However, it is critical to remember that no matter how great one's efforts are, they are not sufficient of themselves to develop the true essence of *bhakti*. It is only by the grace of the Divine, that spiritual devotion is fully manifested:

> *But spiritual devotion is primarily developed from the grace*
> *of the Divine via the blessing of a great Soul.*
> *Bhakti Sutras 38*

There is a great variety among human beings, and due to *karmic* tendencies, spiritual devotion can be developed according to five different attitudes towards the Divine:

- As a servant of the Divine
- As a friend of the Divine
- As a child of the Divine
- As a disciple of the Divine
- As a spouse of the Divine

All five attitudes towards the Divine have their unique aspects, as far as spiritual relationships are concerned, and cannot be judged or rated as better or worse. It would take a separate book to even begin to do justice to the whole subject of spiritual devotion, and all we can do is give a framework for further development.

Traditionally, there are said to be four levels of consciousness in spiritual devotion, and some may say that they are given in order of progressively higher dimensions:

- Worshipful state of consciousness
- Prayerful state of consciousness
- Meditative state of consciousness
- Unified state of consciousness

Until one is fully merged with the Divine, it is always possible to return to a state of confusion and ignorance, and so there is an injunction to follow the *yama-niyama* nexus even after the development of spiritual devotion:

> *Let there be a firm commitment to maintaining an ethical code, even after the development of spiritual devotion. Otherwise, there is the risk of a fall.*
> Bhakti Sutras 12,13

Part 5
Deeper insights into
Yama & Niyama
An Integrated and Interrelated
System of Perfection

Absolute versus Relative application of Yama

Whenever I start to talk about the practice of *yama*, there is always a spirited discussion about whether there are exceptions to the strict application of these moral restraints. Aren't there cases when it is better to lie than tell the truth? What if the truth will hurt someone? However, Patanjali has stated that the self-restraints are universally applicable:

> *These are valid in all spheres, irrespective of birth, place, time and circumstance and constitute the great exercise of will.*
> Yoga Sutra 2.31

There are no exceptions, and any transgressions will have some *karmic* effects. However, this doesn't mean that there are no choices to make – it just means that we have to be more aware of the ramifications of our choices in the subtle realms and not deceive ourselves that good intentions are enough. It is inherently within the normal mental matrix to seek for exceptions and to justify the breaking of "rules and regulations."

It is easier to deal with the absolute application of the individual *yamas* – there are no circumstances in which there would be no karmic consequences from our actions. Let us consider some examples of breaking *ahimsa*:

If one is threatened with bodily harm, should one defend oneself? This would seem like a natural reaction. However, one can choose to do so, and there may not be any social or state condemnation, but there will be negative *karmic* consequences in proportion to the harm done on the transgressor. The best option is to avoid such situations, followed by escaping from such situations with minimal harm. Next, the sages would counsel trying to convince the misguided soul to desist from such negative action. Finally, the only thing left to do would be to suffer the violence from another without retaliation. Such advice of course runs counter to the current culture of macho retaliation, where violence is so often glorified on television, motion pictures and written fiction.

What if we move it around so that someone else is being threatened with bodily harm or even death? Should you defend one person by harming another? Obviously there is good *karma* if you prevent violence being done to that person, but then you are also performing violence in turn – it would naturally be balanced according to spiritual law, but the sages have noted that in most circumstances the perpetuation of violence cannot lead to any permanent positive effects.

However there is a duty for those who can do so, to defend the defenseless. If it is one's dharma to overcome evil-doers, and if one can do so without attachment to the actions performed, then there may be no guilt or negative consequences. Such situations are possible for those tasked with defense of the state or justice, where there can be very little or no consequences, according to the degree of non-attachment. It is very difficult and only a spiritual warrior would be able to achieve this – not those soldiers trained to kill and maim in modern warfare, however noble their intentions may be.

Such analyses are not merely theoretical mental activities. They have to lead to actual change in one's way of life. We must understand the true teachings of these moral restraints to avoid confusion or delusion about the consequences of all actions. Sometimes the "right thing to do" may be too difficult in our current spiritual state, and we may choose a lesser path – there is no condemnation. We just have to be aware of what we are choosing.

Things get even more complicated when we look at situations where there may be an apparent conflict between two *yamas*. There can be many scenarios where non-violence and truth may seem to be a struggle. Should one lie to save a life? Should one tell the truth when it may cost a life? Let us suppose that a friend has committed a heinous crime, and suppose you are opposed to capital punishment. If you lie and save the man's life, then you will be accountable from a *karmic* perspective. In the case where the person has not committed the crime, but has no alibi, and you lie to give the poor soul an alibi, there is still a balancing between the good deed against the lie – it will fall where it will fall.

There is a school of thought called the Way of Action, that proposes the primacy of *ahimsa* over the other *yamas* – that it is okay to lie or steal to save a life. However, this is relative way of thought may no be in full accordance with the teachings of the sages, and one may have to pay the consequences.

Let us look at one more scenario: you live in a totalitarian state which has recently started to persecute an ethnic minority by taking them away en masse. There are reliable reports that they are being secretly exterminated. Some of your best friends are from this minority and you've been surreptitiously helping them with food and medicine. Consequently, you know where a group of them are hiding. After some time, your behavior has raised the suspicions of your neighbors who have reported you to the authorities. The secret police come in the middle of the night and take you away for questioning.

Your choices:

- Tell the truth and reveal the hiding place of your friends and probably result in their death. You subscribe to *satya* or non-lying, but have broken *ahimsa* or non-violence.
- Lie and deny helping the minority or knowing their location. This saves them from harm, but you must take the consequences of lying. The secret police may still hold you or torture you to elicit a change in your testimony.

- Tell the truth that you have helped the minority but refuse to reveal their location. This satisfies both the *yamas* of *ahimsa* and of *satya*, but will surely invite torture or worse suffering.

The sages would counsel the third course of action, as being the most beneficial for spiritual development. However, it may no be particularly pleasant in this life!

Let us all pray for the divine grace that we may not be placed into such difficult moral situations, and if we are so plunged, give us the guidance to take the best course of action.

Discrimination – the key to
Transforming Karma to Dharma

Discrimination is a translation of the Sanskrit term *viveka*, a power of consciousness that leads to liberation from ignorance. It is the innate ability of consciousness to discern the real from the unreal. The continuous application of *viveka* leads to the cessation of the mental afflictions which cause the modifications of consciousness, leading the realization of our Divinve identity, and freedom from the veils of illusion (*maya*). Freedom from the misidentification with the non-self gives freedom from the law of cause and effect or *karma*.

Patanjali has said in his Sutras:

> *The knowledge born of discrimination is liberating, non-sequential and (inclusive) of all conditions and all times.*

This means that discrimination leads to a state, which is not limited by time and space. An act done in the past does not have to play out its consequences any more. The *niyama* of *svadyaya* or self-study helps us to develop this power of *viveka*.

Shankara, in his Crest Jewel of Discrimination points out that in order to achieve Self-Realization and overcome ignorance, the best tool is *viveka*:

> *Neither by weapons, by any scripture, by fire, or by water, can this tree of ignorance be hewn down; nor by millions of different kinds of works can it be hewn down. Only the great sword of discrimination can cut down this Maya, that sword should be whetted by the grace of the Lord.*

Discrimination can be practiced at different levels. In the first stage, it may be as simple as distinguishing what is helpful on the spiritual path, and what can be hindrances, and choosing those that are more helpful. This takes discipline and perseverance, for how often have we rejected what was good for us and went after what we knew in our hearts was "bad" for us?

Discrimination helps us to understand and see the consequences of our thoughts, speech and actions. At every moment, we are free to choose. Do we choose to follow our normal pattern of strengthening the web of desires, by our thoughts, words and deeds, or do we break the cycle of ignorance? Discrimination lets us see the *karmic* consequences of our choices, separating those leading to suffering from those leading to happiness and bliss.

The application of our *viveka h*elps us to distinguish the permanent from the transitory, the real from the relatively real or unreal, the Self from the world. Discrimination is a constant, continuous and focused practice of awareness of the true versus the untrue – the *dharmic* versus the *adharmic*. It is seeng the truth in every situation and acting in accordance with detachment.

At all times, positive or negative circumstances occur around us, due to mutual karmic interactions. By our self-discipline, we determine how we react to these occurences. Through our discrimination, we realize that it is non-productive to hold on to negative emotions, such as anger and violence. Through our practice of *ahimsa* or non-violence, we can react with love instead. Therefore, discrimination works in conjunction with the *yamas*

In an ancient land ruled Jayadeva, a king of the Solar dynasty. He was noted for his wisdom, thoughtfulness and courage. Although a great warrior, he was righteous and peace-loving. During his benevolent rule, the country became prosperous as well the creative leader in arts, literature, music, commerce and philosophy. There was peace in the land as never before.

To ensure the spiritual welfare of his people, he built as many temples as the deities worshiped by them. The splendor of his achievements was unparalleled. The people were contented.

However, as time passed, the king became old but had no heir to follow him. This worried his ministers considerably, but they did not know how to approach the subject. In time the king became more and more inward-looking and spent his time on spiritual pursuits, and it became apparent to his ministers, that he was preparing to transition into the next life. They became desperate and gathered the courage to approach their sovereign.

After paying their respects, the chief minister came forward with folded hands and said, "Majesty, we are greatly distressed and would ask you to solve a dire problem facing our land."

Jayedeva was puzzled, "I am not aware of any serious problem facing our people. What can it be? Tell me and it shall be removed so that you can be at ease once again!"

The wise minister nodded his head and responded, "Lord, your people are happy, contented and have no material or spiritual wants, thanks to your righteous rule. But if you should leave us for the other world, who can we rely on to rule us so ably and efficiently, so justly and judiciously, so lovingly and thoughtfully? Our country has not been blessed with an heir to succeed your Highness. This is the cause of our anxiety."

Jayedeva smiled and said, "My beloved ministers, thank you for bringing this concern to me. I will soon choose my heir, to ensure a smooth transition. My heir will be a just and wise ruler with great discrimination and single-minded in his love for the people." This reply surprised the ministers for they knew it was no easy task to choose a worthy heir for their unparalleled king, but they had faith in his judgment and waited for the drama to unfold.

The king soon gave his ministers detailed instructions for the organization and building of a huge carnival, the size of a town. He architected the layout and types of attractions to be displayed and the games to be played. He then asked his ministers to go and announce to the people that he was giving them a chance to show their determination and discrimination. Somewhere in the carnival, in the center of attraction, was a place he had chosen to stay in. The person who recognizes him and identifies him in the carnival would be chosen as his heir.

The wise king had designed the stalls and booths to be very tempting and distracting for the people, so that only the strong-willed, persevering and discriminating individual would be capable of identifying him, in the middle of so many attractions.

On entering the carnival, people became mesmerized by the number and variety of stalls, booths and performances. There were lotteries, shooting galleries, burlesque shows, comedy and magic shows, swimming pools, performing animals, arts and crafts galore from all over the world, the tasty food stalls satisfying the palate of one and all, and many other items of display. The carnival ground was resplendent in displays of banners, flags and streamers. The place provided fun, frolic and mirth not only to the young but also to the old. There was even a temple built in one corner, with a large tank filled with crystal clear water. No one who entered wished to leave this carnival.

The carnival was opened day and night and never closed, and would operate until the heir was chosen. Tens of thousands of people from all over the country came to see the magnificent carnival. The stalls were alluring, the booths enticing, the dancing halls tempting and the theatres enthralling. Caught up in such attractions people forgot that they had gone there to identify the king and thereby become the heir. Some who had a degree of patience, tried to see if they could identify the king in any of the people stationed in the stalls. So strenuous was this task that in the end they gave it up and took to enjoying the objects displayed instead.

Many days passed and then came a young knight riding a horse from a neighboring town. He decided not to waste his time by walking and so rode on horseback into the carnival with the single aim of finding the king.

With his subtle mind he examined the sights that he saw and applied his discriminative faculty to separate the revelers and performers. Although his mind was yoked to the goal of identifying the king, he did not despise the sights that he saw nor the sweet melodies that he heard. Outwardly he seemed to enjoy everything that came his way with a smile and a nod of his head, but his keen and incisive intellect was trying to separate the illusive carnival play from the reality of royalty.

After some time, even he seemed to lose heart, for in vain had he searched in all the likely places. However, in his innermost heart of hearts, the yearning for the goal sustained him, releasing an extra spurt of energy overcoming his disappointment. Finally he came to the temple, the only place he had not yet searched. To purify himself, he had a bath in the temple-tank, and with reverence entered the temple, going straight to the holy of holies, the inner sanctum. There he had a vision of the deity of his heart, but not the presence of the king.

The young man than applied his contemplative discrimination. It felt right that the king would be found in the temple, but the knight failed to find any trace of him, even after going around the temple three times. His mind became quiescent and he stood apart and in a flash had a vision of the king seated in a room behind a secret passage. Immediately, he examined the walls of the inner sanctum and saw a carved block of stone which projected slightly more than rest. He had to use all of his strength to pull on it, but slowly it came out. Behind the stone, the resolute young man saw a secret passage. It was dark, but he stepped into the darkness feeling his way with his hands. Soon he came to another stone-structure, with a projecting square block. Lifting it, he slid it down the wall.

A blinding white light streamed out from a beautifully decorated chamber. The smiling king was seated on a golden throne in the centre of the carpeted floor and jeweled ceiling. After his long search, the young knight was speechless at the magnificence of the Lord of his Land. He prostrated himself before the king paying his respects. The king too felt happy, for the Divine Maker had ushered into his presence a worthy heir.

This world with its myriad attractions and distractions is the Carnival of Life. The Divine Creator is the ruler Jayadeva. He has sent us into the world not only to enjoy its beauties but also to recognize that we soon lose our identification with the Supreme, when immersed in the attractions of the world of objects, emotions and thoughts.

We can only realize our True Self if we act like the young knight and apply our discriminative faculties with perseverance, to unravel the real from the unreal. We should not allow the objects of the senses to entice us away from our unity with the Divine, but at the same time we need not despise the world of objects. We can enjoy everything that comes our way, but should not become slaves of enjoyment, constantly applying the self-discipline of the *niyama* to develop our discrimination and our self-restraint or *yama* to ensure proper actions.

The practice of the eight limbs of Yoga, is the process by which the impurities dwindle away and there dawns the light of wisdom leading to discriminative discernment.

In the early stages, the development of discrimination may actually give rise to fear and disillusion with ordinary experience. This is because we start to see that everything we used to think of as real and importanf for our happiness, is turning out to be unreal and unimportant. Such a reversal of our norma way of thinking can be a difficult transition, jus as growing up can be:

To the people who have developed discrimination, all is misery on account of the pains resulting from change, anxiety and tendencies, as also on account of the conflicts between the functioning for the gunas and the vrittis of the mind.

After the stage of fear and disillusion, discrimination gives rise to the light of spiritual illumination, which guides the aspirant through the path. By the continuous awareness of reality, ignorance is overcome, and the emergence of new *karma* is prevented. Finally in conjunction with *vairagya*, or non-attachment, the state of *dharma-megha-samadhi* is realized, and the seeds of previous *karmas* are "burnt" away.

The "unceasing vision of discernment" according to the sages is achieved when there is total identification with the Self in *asmaprajnatah samadhi*. The process is meditative awareness of the Self, leading to absorption, leading to complete identification.

It is well to keep in mind that due to the *karmic* results of past actions, it is difficult ot disengage from the external world, by even strong meditative practices. As long as one feels pleasure and pain, so long *karma* remains, and only the knowledge of "atman brahma" does away with all past actions done in countless number of births. Discrimination is the ability to discern the real from the unreal. It is only by means of discrimination that doubt of whatever kind may be excluded. There are no circumstances where the aspirant should fail to see the one reality underlying all, to find the "king" hidden in the Carnival of Life.

Jesus the Jewish Yogi

A great *yogi* and teacher called Jesus walked the earth two thousand years ago. The sum and total of his external teachings which have been handed down in the New Testament, is the practice of *yamas* and *niyamas* for the purification and transformation of the human mind.

It would be superfluous of me to recount his life for it has been dramatized countless times in all kinds of media. A great portion of the world took to Jesus for guidance, but hardly any follow his instructions.

Chapter 5 of the book of Matthew gives concise summary of the program of practice that Jesus advised for humanity. Before we read his inspiring words, it is instructive to remember that he practiced the *tapas* of fasting to build up the internal spiritual fire before overcoming his negative tendencies:

> *Then Jesus was lead up by the Spirit into the wilderness to be tempted by the devil. And when he had fasted forty days and forty nights, afterward he was hungry.*
> *Matthew 4:1-2*

The teachings

When he saw the crowds, he went up the mountain, and after he had sat down, his disciples came to him.

He began to teach them, saying:

Blessed are the poor in spirit, for theirs is the kingdom of heaven.
[refer the *yama* of non-attachment or *aparigraha*]

Blessed are they who mourn, for they will be comforted.

Blessed are the meek, for they will inherit the land.

Blessed are they who hunger and thirst for righteousness, for they will be satisfied.

Blessed are the merciful, for they will be shown mercy. [**consider the *yama* of *ahimsa***]

Blessed are the pure of heart, for they will see God. [*refer niyama of* purity *or saucha*]

Blessed are the peacemakers, for they will be called children of God.

Blessed are they who are persecuted for the sake of righteousness, for theirs is the kingdom of heaven. [**refer the *yama* of *satya* or truth**]

Blessed are you when they insult you and persecute you and utter every kind of evil against you (falsely) because of me.

Rejoice and be glad, for your reward will be great in heaven. Thus they persecuted the prophets who were before you.

You are the salt of the earth. But if salt loses its taste, with what can it be seasoned? It is no longer good for anything but to be thrown out and trampled underfoot.

You are the light of the world. A city set on a mountain cannot be hidden.

Nor do they light a lamp and then put it under a bushel basket; it is set on a lamp-stand, where it gives light to all in the house. Just so, your light must shine before others, that they may see your good deeds and glorify your heavenly Father.

Do not think that I have come to abolish the law or the prophets. I have come not to abolish but to fulfill.

Amen, I say to you, until heaven and earth pass away, not the smallest letter or the smallest part of a letter will pass from the law, until all things have taken place.

Therefore, whoever breaks one of the least of these commandments and teaches others to do so will be called least in the kingdom of heaven. But whoever obeys and teaches these commandments will be called greatest in the kingdom of heaven. [**Jesus was no supporter of the relative application of the moral restraints**]

I tell you, unless your righteousness surpasses that of the scribes and Pharisees, you will not enter into the kingdom of heaven.

You have heard that it was said to your ancestors, 'You shall not kill; and whoever kills will be liable to judgment.

But I say to you, whoever is angry with his brother will be liable to judgment, and whoever says to his brother, "Raca," will be answerable to the Council, and whoever says, "You fool," will be in danger of hell fire. [**a very strong statement for verbal** *ahimsa*]

Therefore, if you bring your gift to the altar, and there recall that your brother has anything against you, leave your gift there at the altar, go first and be reconciled with your brother, and then come and offer your gift.

Settle with your opponent quickly while on the way to court with him. Otherwise your opponent will hand you over to the judge, and the judge will hand you over to the guard, and you will be thrown into prison.

Amen, I say to you, you will not be released until you have paid the last penny. [Jesus taught the law of *Karma*]

You have heard that it was said, 'You shall not commit adultery.'

But I say to you, everyone who looks at a woman with lust has already committed adultery with her in his heart.

If your right eye causes you to sin, tear it out and throw it away. It is better for you to lose one of your members than to have your whole body thrown into hell fire.

And if your right hand causes you to sin, cut it off and throw it away. It is better for you to lose one of your members than to have your whole body go into hell fire.

It was also said, 'Whoever divorces his wife must give her a bill of divorce.'

But I say to you, whoever divorces his wife (unless the marriage is unlawful) causes her to commit adultery, and whoever marries a divorced woman commits adultery.

Again you have heard that it was said to your ancestors, 'Do not take a false oath, but make good to the Lord all that you vow.'

But I say to you, do not swear at all; not by heaven, for it is God's throne; nor by the earth, for it is his footstool; nor by Jerusalem, for it is the city of the great King.

Do not swear by your head, for you cannot make a single hair white or black.

Let your 'Yes' mean 'Yes,' and your 'No' mean 'No.' Anything more is from the evil one. [**a concise solution for** *satya* **or non-lying**]

You have heard that it was said, 'An eye for an eye and a tooth for a tooth.'

But I say to you, offer no resistance to one who is evil. When someone strikes you on (your) right cheek, turn the other one to him as well.

If anyone wants to go to law with you over your tunic, hand him your cloak as well.

Should anyone press you into service for one mile, go with him for two miles.

Give to the one who asks of you, and do not turn your back on one who wants to borrow.

You have heard that it was said, 'You shall love your neighbor and hate your enemy.'

But I say to you, love your enemies, and pray for those who persecute you, that you may be children of your heavenly Father, for he makes his sun rise on the bad and the good, and causes rain to fall on the just and the unjust. For if you love those who love you, what recompense will you have? Do not the tax collectors do the same? And if you greet your brothers only, what is unusual about that? Do not the non-believers do the same? [**Love as the ultimate expression of *ahimsa***]

So be perfect, just as your heavenly Father is perfect. [**the goal of Yoga**]

Another great *yogic* teaching from Jesus is the distillation of the *niyamas* into a simple prayer, easy to learn and inspiring to all who have had the good fortune to know it: The Lord's Prayer.

The Lord's Prayer

Jesus, the Christ taught his disciples the Lord's Prayer, in Matthew 6.9, and illustrated that the principles of the *niyama* transcend religious boundaries:

Our Father who is in Heaven
Hallowed be your Name, your kingdom come.
The culmination of *svadyaya* or self-study is the realization of the truth of relationship between divinity and humanity. Jesus studied the scriptures and learnt from the wise men of his day, even traveling to far off places like Egypt and India (according to *yogic* tradition).

Your will be done on earth as it is in heaven.
The direct realization of divinity leads to *ishvar prandhan* or total surrender to the divine will.

Give us this day our daily bread.
A state of contentment or *santosha*.

Forgive us our trespasses, as we forgive those who trespass against us.
In the state of *saucha* or purity, love transcends all enmity. Jesus also taught the golden rule: Do to others as you would others do to you. Since one would normally not do violence to one-self, this is the rule for *ahimsa* or nonviolence.

And lead us not into temptation, but deliver us from evil.
By the development of *tapas* or inner spiritual fire, all negativities are burnt.

Amen.
Let the path lead to the goal.

Yamas and Ethics

We've explored and practiced the moral restraints of *yamas* based on the principles of *dharma* and *karma*. From the yogic perspective, these so-called moral injunctions are a necessary part of achieving Self-Realization. They are the way that a self-realized *yogi* would act. Their basis is the experience and insight of those who've reached the goal and overcome the darkness of ignorance.

It can also be instructive to examine how the field of ethics can be formulated in the absence of the spiritual law of *karma*, as in the Western Philosophy.

Ethics is also called moral philosophy – consisting of the conceptual systematization of right and wrong behavior. Philosophers today usually divide the field of Ethics into three general areas:

- Meta-ethics tries to deal with where ethical principles come from, and what they mean – whether they are merely social inventions or only expressions of our individual emotions or actually based on universal truths. How does the will of God or the role of individual reason in ethical judgments factor into these principles?
- Normative ethics takes on the task of providing a system of moral standards that regulate right and wrong conduct. This involves postulating the good habits that we should acquire, the duties that we should follow, or the consequences of our behavior on others.
- Applied ethics involves examining specific controversial issues, such as euthanasia, abortion, homosexuality or capital punishment. For example, the issue of abortion is an applied ethical topic since it involves a specific type of controversial behavior, but it also depends normative principles, such as the right of self-rule and the right to life, which are litmus tests for determining the morality of that

procedure. The issue also rests on meta-ethical issues such as, "where do rights come from?" and "what kind of beings have rights?"

We will restrict our focus on the topic of normative ethics, as it tries to justify specific systems of moral behavior.

Normative Ethics

The Golden Rule is a classic example of a normative principle: We should do to others what we would want others to do to us. Since I do not want my neighbor to steal my car, then it is wrong for me to steal her car. Since I would want people to feed me if I was starving, then I should help feed starving people. Using this same reasoning, we can theoretically determine whether any possible action is right or wrong. So, based on the Golden Rule, it would also be wrong for me to lie to, harass, victimize, assault, or kill others. The Golden Rule is an example of a normative theory that establishes a single principle against which we judge all actions. Other normative theories are based a set of foundational principles, or a set of good character traits. The key assumption in normative ethics is that there is only one ultimate criterion of moral conduct, whether it is a single rule or a set of principles.

There are three primary ethical strategies: (1) virtue-based, (2) duty-based, and (3) consequence-based.

Virtue-based Ethics

Instead of following precisely defined rules of conduct, such as "don't kill" or "don't steal," virtue theorists place the emphasis on the importance of developing good habits of character, such as benevolence. Once you've acquired benevolence you'll then habitually act in a benevolent manner. Plato emphasized four virtues in particular, which were later called cardinal virtues: wisdom, courage, temperance and justice. Other classic virtues are fortitude, generosity, self-respect, good temper, and sincerity. Christians emphasized the virtues of faith, hope and charity. Of course, the counterbalance is that we should avoid acquiring bad character traits such as cowardice, injustice, and vanity. Virtue theory emphasizes moral education it is the responsibility of the adults in society and family to instill virtues in the young.

After analyzing some specific virtues, Aristotle realized that most virtues fall at a mean between more extreme character traits. For example, if one does not have enough courage, there is a tendency towards cowardice, which is a vice. On the other hand, if one has too much courage there is a tendency towards rashness which is also a vice. Therefore it necessary to enlist the aid of reason to find the perfect mean between extreme character traits.

Duty-based Ethics

These are based on the realization that we feel clear obligations or duties as human beings, such as caring for our young, and not to commit murder. Such duties are irrespective of the consequences that might follow from our actions - it is wrong to neglect our children even if it results in some great benefit, such as financial savings. There are three main duty theories:

German philosopher S. Pufendorf classified dozens of duties under three headings: duties to God, duties to oneself, and duties to others.
- There are two kinds of duties towards God: a duty to know the existence and nature of God and a practical duty to both inwardly and outwardly worship God.
- There are two kinds of duties towards oneself: duties of the soul, which involve developing one's skills and talents,

and duties of the body, which involve not harming our bodies, such as through gluttony, drunkenness or suicide.

- Our duties towards others can be divided into absolute duties, which are universally binding on people, and conditional duties, which are the result of contracts between people. Absolute duties are of three sorts: avoid wronging others, treating others as equals, and promoting the good of others. Conditional duties involve various types of contracts or agreements, such as the duty is to keep one's promises.

A second duty-based approach to Ethics is called the rights theory. The British philosopher John Locke argued that the laws of nature mandate that we should not harm anyone's life, health, liberty or possessions - these are our natural rights, given to us by God. Following Locke, the United States Declaration of Independence authored by Thomas Jefferson recognized three foundational rights: life, liberty, and the pursuit of happiness. Rights theorists maintain that we can deduce more specific rights from these general ones, including the rights of property, movement, speech, and religious expression. There are four distinctive features associated with moral rights: first, rights are natural insofar as they are not invented or created by governments; second, they are universal, that is they do not change from country to country; third, they are equal in the sense that rights are the same for all people, irrespective of gender, race, or handicap; and fourth, they are inalienable which means that one cannot hand over one's rights to another person, such as by selling oneself into slavery.

A third duty-based theory is that by Kant, which emphasizes a single principle of duty that he called the "categorical imperative." – a categorical imperative simply mandates an action, irrespective of one's personal desires, such as "You ought to do X," not because of any desire or need fulfillment, but because it is inherently correct. Kant gave at least four versions of the categorical imperative, but one is especially direct: *Treat people as an end, and never as a means to an end*. Translating this into action means that we should always treat people with dignity, and never use them as mere instruments. For Kant, we treat people as an end whenever our actions toward someone reflect the inherent value of that person. Donating to charity, for example, is morally correct since this acknowledges the inherent value of the recipient. By contrast, we treat someone as a means to an end whenever we treat that person as a tool to achieve something else. It would be wrong, for example, to steal my neighbor's car because I would be treating him as a means to my own happiness. The categorical imperative also regulates the morality of actions that affect us individually. Suicide, for example, would be wrong since one would be treating one's life as a means to the alleviation of one's misery. Kant believed that the morality of all actions could be determined by appealing to this single principle of duty.

Consequence-based Ethics

According to consequence-based normative theories, correct moral conduct is determined solely by a cost-benefit analysis of an action's consequences: An action is morally right if the consequences of that action are more favorable than unfavorable.

This form of Ethics requires that we first tally both the good and bad consequences of an action, and then determine whether the total good consequences outweigh the total bad consequences. If the good consequences are greater, then the action is morally proper. If the bad consequences are greater, then the action is morally improper.

In the 18th century philosophers wanted a quick way to morally assess an action by appealing to experience, rather than by appealing to feelings or long lists of duties. There are three different consequential perspectives:

- Ethical Egoism: an action is morally right if the consequences of that action are more favorable than unfavorable only to the agent performing the action.

- Ethical Altruism: an action is morally right if the consequences of that action are more favorable than unfavorable to everyone except the agent.

- Utilitarianism: an action is morally right if the consequences of that action are more favorable than unfavorable to everyone.

Thomas Hobbes, developed a social contract theory based on ethical egoism - for purely selfish reasons, everyone is better off living in a world with moral rules than one without moral rules. For without moral rules, we are subject to the whims of other people's selfish interests. Our property, our families, and even our lives are at continual risk. Selfishness alone will therefore motivate everyone to adopt a basic set of rules which will allow for a civilized community. Not surprisingly, these rules would include prohibitions against lying, stealing and killing. However, these rules will ensure safety for each agent only if the rules are enforced. As selfish creatures, each of us would plunder our neighbors' property once their guards were down. Each agent would then be at risk from his neighbor. Therefore, for selfish reasons alone, we devise a means of enforcing these rules: we create a policing agency which punishes us if we violate these rules.

All three of these theories focus on the consequences of actions for different groups of people and therefore will yield different conclusions. An often cited example: A person was traveling through a developing country when he witnessed a car in front of him run off the road and roll over several times. He asked the hired driver to pull over to assist, but, to his surprise, the driver accelerated nervously past the scene. After going a sage distance, the driver explain that that country if someone assists an accident victim, then the police often hold the assisting person responsible for the accident itself. If the victim dies, then the assisting person could be held responsible for the death. Consequently, road accident victims are therefore usually left unattended and often die from exposure to the country's harsh desert conditions.

On the principle of ethical egoism, the person would only be concerned with the consequences to him if he offered assistance - the decision to drive on would be the morally proper choice. On the principle of ethical altruism, one would be concerned only with the consequences of the action as others are affected, particularly the accident victim - assisting the victim would be the morally correct choice, irrespective of the negative consequences that result for him. On the principle of utilitarianism, he must consider the consequences for both himself and the victim - the outcome here is less clear, and there would need to be a precise calculation of the overall benefit versus dis-benefit of stopping to help.

Utilitarianism can get very complicated and would need some sort of moral super-accountant to figure out. Many ways of calculating benefits have been proposed:

- Act-utilitarianism: tally the consequences of each action we perform and thereby determine on a case by case basis whether an action is morally right or wrong. The problem with this is that universally reprehensible acts such as torture and slavery could be justified if the social benefits could be shown to outweigh the negative affects!
- Hedonistic utilitarianism: tally the pleasure and pain which results from our actions. The issue is that not all moral choices can be boiled down to pleasure and pain principles.
- Rule-utilitarianism: a behavioral code or rule is morally right if the consequences of adopting that rule are more favorable than unfavorable to everyone. Unlike act utilitarianism, which weighs the consequences of each particular action,

rule-utilitarianism offers a litmus test only for the morality of moral rules, such as "stealing is wrong." Adopting a rule against theft clearly has more favorable consequences than unfavorable consequences for everyone. The same is true for moral rules against lying or murdering.

It is hoped that this brief excursion into the mire of Ethics can give the spiritual seeker great relief to return to the relatively simpler *karmic* based *yamas*.

Yama, Niyama & Ashtanga Yoga

It is not by chance that the *yogic* sage Patanjali has placed *ahimsa* as the first of the *yama*. Non-violence is the most important practice to perform – it leads to the perfection of love. It is the most practical to practice because it is very easy to observe whether one has broken the self-restraint in action, speech or thought. The perfection of love removes the veil of duality and ignorance, merging into *satya* or truth – the highest aspect of which is the realization of the essential one-ness of all Being. With the perfection of *satya*, all covetousness is removed and non-stealing or *asteya* happens in due course. The ultimate in stealing is the thought of keeping something away from the Divine, the giver and owner of all there is. With the perfection of *asteya*, all that we have is offered to the Divine, which is what *brahmacharya* is all about – the turning of all our energies toward the Divine. When we have given our all back to the Source of All, what is there to be attached to anymore? The perfection of *brahmacharya* leads effortlessly to the practice of *aparigraha* or non-attachment.

Although I've presented the *yamas* as a progression, one leading to the next in perfection, this does not mean that the spiritual seeker needs to wait for the perfection of one before practicing the next. They should all be practiced in unison as a completely integrated way of life. However, each cannot be perfected until the previous one has been perfected first, and therefore *ahimsa* is the most important one to work towards.

When the *yamas* are perfected, there is an emergence of *saucha* or purity, the first of the *niyamas*. The purpose of the self-restraints is to provide the ground for purity and by perfecting purity, all thoughts, words and deeds become sanctified and will no longer incur new *karmic* consequences. With the perfection of purity, contentment or *santosha* arises in consequence. You might now start to wonder how contentment could possibly lead to austerity.

It is well to recall that *tapas* is actually the development of inner fire, and this inner fire requires the quenching of all desires, which can only occur when contentment is perfected. When the inner fire has developed by burning all the desires, it is then possible to realize one's true Self, and *svadhyaya* becomes a reality. With the perfection of *svadhyaya*, one can truly surrender to the will of the Divine and practice the perfection of *ishvar pranidhana*.

Again, the *niyamas* are a natural progression from the *yamas*, and each *niyama* smoothly merges into the next.

The third *anga* of Ashtanga Yoga, after *niyama*, is *pranayama*, the control and expansion of the life-force energy. This *pranayama* is a practice of combining the *tapas* or building of inner fire, done with self-awareness of *svadhyaya* and with devotion to the Divine, in a state of *ishvar pranidhana*. By the continuous and prolonged practice of *pranayama*, the state of *pratyahara* or the internalization of the senses comes about. It is important to remember that *pratyahara* is the consequence of the consistent practice of life-force control. The deepening of *pratyahara* leads to *dharana* or one-pointed concentration, which leads to *dhyana* or meditative awareness, which leads to *samadhi*, states of blissful absorption into the Self and eventually the Divine. Each limb of Ashtanga Yoga flowers into the next, as opening blossoms encouraging the growth of the next higher lotus bloom.

Yoga is not possible without the fragrance of the *yama* and *niyama*, the their purifying and transformative power. Let us firmly make our progress on the spiritual path by building the strong foundation of self-restraint and self-discipline.

Recommended Reading

Gandhi, M.K.: Non-Violence. New Directions Publishing. 1965.

Gandhi, M.K.: The Bhagvadgita. Orient Paperbacks. 8th printing. 1998.

Taimni, I.K.: The Science of Yoga. Quest Books. 7th printing. 1992.

Duggal, K.S.(Compiled & Translated): Guru Nanak. UBSPD. 1997.

King, Martin Luther: Stride toward Freedom. Harper. 1958.

Francis of Assisi: The Best from all his Works. Thomas Nelson Inc. 1989.

Muruganar, Sri: The Garland of Guru's Sayings [the collection of Ramana Maharshi's answers to spiritual seekers]. V.S. Ramanan. 1990.

Prakesh, Prem: The Yoga of Spiritual Devotion [A modern translation of the Narada Bhakti Sutras]. Inner Traditions. 1998.

Glossary

A

Adharma. A lack of virtue or righteousness

Adrishta. The impelling, unseen power of one's own past actions

Agni. The cosmic Fire element

Ahamkara. The 'I-maker' - the individuation principle, or ego, which must be transcended for Self-realization

Ahimsa. Non-harming – an important moral discipline (*yama*)

Ajna Chakra. Third-eye; sixth energy center, in the center of the head

Akasha. Ether/space - the first of the five material elements of which the physical universe is composed

Anahata Chakra. Heart center; the fifth energy center

Ananda. Bliss - the state of utter joy, which is an essential quality of the ultimate Reality

Apana. Aspect of life-force energy in the body, functioning in excretion

Apas. The cosmic Water element

Asana. Seat - a physical posture; originally this meant only a meditation posture, but has subsequently been greatly developed in Hatha Yoga

Ashtanga. The eight-limbed comprehensive yogic system

Atman. Self - the true Self, or Spirit, which is eternal and super-conscious

Avatar. A divine incarnation, such as Rama, Krishna from Vishnu, and Babaji from Shiva

Avidya. Ignorance - the root cause of suffering (*duhkha*)

B

Babaji. Immortal being responsible for the spiritual evolution of mankind. He works in the background, without interfering with the free-will of humanity. See also *Gorakshanath*. *Babaji* is the Ancient of Days. He was first brought to the notice of the West in *Yogananda's* classic, 'Autobiography of a Yogi'

Bandha. A physical lock in yogic postures

Bhakta. Devotee - a disciple practicing *Bhakti-Yoga*
Bhakti. Devotion - the love of the devotee toward the Divine or the *guru*
Bhastrika. A type of purifying breath control exercise
Bhuta Shuddhi. Purification of the five elements which constitute the physical and subtle bodies
Bija. A seed or source
Brahma. The Divine principle of Creation; Creator of the universe
Brahmacharya. The discipline of chastity, which produces *ojas*
Buddha. The 'awakened one' - designation of the person who has attained enlightenment; title of *Gautama*, the historic founder of Buddhism, who lived in the sixth century B.C.E.
Buddhi. Intellect; understanding, reason; light of consciousness

C
Chakra. Wheel - one of the psycho-energetic centers of the subtle body
Cit. Consciousness; the super-conscious ultimate Reality
Chitta. Mind-stuff; mental substratum

D
Deva. The shining one - a male deity or a high angelic being
Devi. She who shines - a female deity or a high angelic being
Dharma. Law – right conduct
Dhyana. Meditation
Diksha. A transfer of wisdom or power through initiation
Dosha. A fault; the categories of physical constitution in the medical system of *Ayurveda*

G
Goraksha. Lord of the senses ['protector of cows'] - the Immortal founder of *Hatha-Yoga*; disciple of *Matsyendranath*. See also *Gorakshanath* and *Babaji*
Gorakshanath. The formal designation for *Goraksha*, as the founder of the *Nath Sampradaya*, the ancient upholders of *Yoga*

Guna. The fundamental building blocks of nature expressed as a triad of brightness, activity and inertia

Guru. A spiritual teacher; *acarya*; literally, "he who is heavy, weighty"

H

Hamsa. Swan – the Soul; particularly for that which is being propelled by the breath

Hatha-Yoga. A major branch of Yoga, developed by *Gorakshanath*; Ha-tha is the union of the sun and moon; with emphasis on the energetic and physical tools of transformation, such as postures, cleansing techniques, and breath control

I

Ida-nadi. The energy or *prâna* current on the left side of the central channel (*sushumna-nadi*) associated with the parasympathetic nervous system and having a cooling or calming effect on the mind when activated

Ishvara-pranidhana. Dedication to the Lord – surrender to the will of the Divine; one of the *Niyamas*, or *Ashtanga*

J

Japa. The recitation of *mantras*

Jivatman. The 'individual self' as opposed to the ultimate Self (*parama-âtman*)

Jivan-mukta. A Siddha who, while still embodied, has attained liberation (*moksha*)

Jnana. Knowledge/wisdom

K

Kaivalya. The state of absolute freedom from conditioned existence

Kama. Desire - the appetite for sensual pleasure blocking the path to true bliss (*ananda*)

Kapalabhati. A rapid breathing technique for purification of the energy body

Kapha. One of the doshas; predominance of Water element in the physical body constitution

Karma. Activity of any kind; the law of *karma* is the law of causation

Kevala kumbakha. Spontaneous cessation of breath

Khecari-mudra. The Hatha Yoga practice of curling the tongue back against the upper palate in order to seal the life energy (*prana*)

Kosha. Any one of five "envelopes" surrounding the true Self (*atman*) and thus blocking its light – the physical body is called *annamayakosha* ['envelope made of food']

Krishna. An incarnation of God Vishnu, the God-man whose teachings can be found in the *Bhagavad-Gita*

Kriya Yoga. An evolutionary practice for Self Realization, founded by Babaji

Kumbhaka. Breath retention; a part of *Pranayama*

Kundalini-shakti. The spiritual energy, which exists in potential form at the lowest psycho-energetic center of the body [*muladhara chakra*) and which must be awakened and guided to the center at the crown (*sahasrara chakra*) for Self Realization

M

Mahamudra. Great Seal. A practice of importance in Kriya Yoga

Manas. Mind - the lower mind, which is bound to the senses

Manipura chakra. The navel or third energy center

Mantra. A sacred sound or phrase, such as *om*, with a transforming effect on the mind of the individual reciting it; to be ultimately effective, a *mantra* needs to be given in an initiatory context (*dīkshâ*)

Matsyendranath. 'Lord of Fish' - Guru of Gorakshanath; a great Yogi, remembered by the Buddhists as Avalokiteshwara, the Boddhisatva of Compassion

Maya. Illusion by which the world is seen as separate from the ultimate Reality

Moksha. Release / Liberation - the condition of freedom from ignorance (*avidya*) and the binding effect of *karma*

N

Nadi. Energy Channel – there are 72,000 subtle channels through which the life force (*prana*) circulates

Nadi Shodana. Purification of the energy channels

Nadi Shuddhi. Purification of the energy channels

Nath. Lord – the Masters of Yoga

Nath Sampradaya. The tradition flowing through the mists of time, of the Lords of Yoga

Nauli. Abdominal churning exercise

Nirguna. The Eternal Reality beyond all qualities

Niyama. Self-restraint - the second limb of *Ashtanga*, which consists of purity (*shauca*), contentment (*samtosha*), austerity (*tapas*), study (*svadhyaya*), and dedication to the Lord (*ishvara-pranidhana*)

O

Ojas. Vitality - the subtle spiritual energy produced from sexual energy through practice

Om — the original *mantra* symbolizing the ultimate Reality

P

Papa. Negative results caused by desire and ego-centeredness - eliminated when wisdom arises

Paramatman. Supreme self - the truel Self, which is one, as opposed to the plurality of individuated self (*jiva-atman*) existing in the form of living beings

Paramahamsa. Supreme swan – the state of a being, between liberation and Siddhahood

Pingala-nadi. The channel of the *prâna* or life-energy on the right side of the central channel (*sushumna-nadi*) and associated with the sympathetic nervous system and having an energizing effect on the mind when activated

Pitta. One of the *doshas*; a dominance of the Fire element in the physical constitution

Prakriti. Nature, which is unconscious or *acit*

Prana. Life-force sustaining the body; the breath as an external manifestation of the subtle life-force

Pranayama. Breath control - from *prana* and *ayama* - life/breath extension")

Pratyahara. Internalization of the senses; the fifth limb in Ashtanga

Prithvi. The cosmic Earth element

Punya. Merit from righteous and moral action

Purakha. Inhalation phase of breathing

Purusha. The true Self (*atman*) or Spirit

R

Raja-Yoga. ("Royal Yoga") — a late medieval designation of *Patanjali's* eightfold *yoga-darshana,* also known as Classical Yoga, or Ashtanga

Rajas. One of the three Gunas; principle of activity and movement

Rama — an incarnation of God *Vishnu* preceding *Krishna*; the principal hero of the *Ramayana*

Rishi. Cosmic Seer – particularly apt for the Seven *Rishis*, who have ascended to the stars to help cosmic evolution

S

Sadhana. Spiritual discipline or practice leading to perfection

Saguna Brahman. The phenomenal aspect of the Divine

Sahaja. The *sahaja* state is the natural condition, that is, enlightenment or realization

Sahasrara Chakra. The crown or seventh energy center

Samadhi. The state of Yoga; the ecstatic unitive state; there are many types of *samadhi - samprajnâta* (with object), *asamprajnâta* (objectless) and *sahaja*(natural state of enlightenment)

Samsara. The finite world of change, as opposed to the ultimate Reality

Samskara. The subconscious impression left behind by each will-full act, which leads to habitual reactions

Sanatana Dharma. The Eternal Teachings of the sages and yogis

Sat. Being/truth - the ultimate Reality

Sat-Guru. The Guru of Truth – capable of giving the disciple the experience of super-consciousness

Satsang. Company of Truth – being in the company of a Master of Yoga

Sattva. One of the three *gunas*; the principle of light

Shakti. Energy - the dynamic aspect of the Divine; depicted as feminine

Shaktipat. Descent of energy – the transmission of spiritual energy from a Sat-Guru, to speed up the process of Self Realization in the disciple

Shambavi. A concentration technique with eyes, open and focused on the third-eye

Shishya. Student/disciple - the initiated disciple of a *guru*

Shiva. The Auspicious One – the supreme liberating aspect of the Divine; the supreme Yogi

Shuddhi. Purification

Siddha. Perfected Being

Surya. One of the names of our Sun, the highest visible manifestation of the Creative aspect of the Divine

Sushumna-nadi. The central *prâna* or life-force channel counterpart to the physical spinal cord; the *kundalini-shakti* ascends this channel during Self Realization

T

Tapas. Austerity; the fire, heat and light from *sadhana*

Tamas. One of the three *gunas*; the principle of inertia and ignorance

U

Udana. One of the aspect of the life-force energy

V

Vairagya. The abandonment of all passions

Vayu. Air; another term used for the aspects of *prana*

Vata. One of the *doshas*; a predominance of the Air element in the body

Vedanta. The primary non-dualistic metaphysical approach to reality based on the teachings of the Vedas and Upanishads

Vidya. Knowledge/wisdom

Vishnu. The preserver - the aspect of the Divine which has had in this cycle, nine incarnations, including *Rama* and *Krishna*; the tenth incarnation *(avatar) Kalki* is coming at the close of the *kali-yuga*

Vishuddha Chakra. The throat or fifth energy center

Viveka. Discernment or discriminating aspect of wisdom

Vritti. The waves of mental disturbance

Vyana. One of the aspects of the life-force energy; the *prana* which pervades the body

Y

Yajna. Sacrifice; Yoga is an inner sacrifice through meditation and self-surrender

Yoga. The state of Union with the Divine; the path of discipline and practice to achieve Self Realization

Yogi. A Self-Realized Being; commonly used also for a practitioner of Yoga, who has not yet achieved the goal

About the Author

 Rudra Shivananda is dedicated to the service of humanity through the furthering of human awareness and spiritual evolution. He teaches that the only lasting way to bring happiness into one's life is by a consistent practice of awareness and transformation.

 Rudra Shivananda is committed to spreading the message of the immortal Being called *Babaji*. He teaches the message of World and Individual Peace through the practice of *Kriya Yoga*. As a student and teacher of yoga for almost 30 years, he is trained as an *Acharya* or Spiritual Preceptor in the Indian *Nath* Tradition, closely associated with the *Siddha* tradition. He is also a member of *Babaji's Kriya Yoga* Order of *Acharyas* as well as a *Shakti* Healer with expertise in the healing and spiritual uses of gemstones and essential oils. He lives and works in the San Francisco Bay area, and has given initiations and workshops in California, Colorado, Washington, Pennsylvania, Hawaii, Ireland, India, England and Spain.

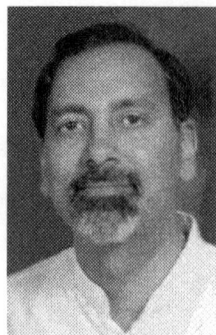

Other books from Alight Publications

Breathe Like Your Life Depends On It
Author: *Rudra Shivananda*
Explore the secrets of Life-force control and expansion for self-Healing, strength and vitality. Imagine living a life protected from stress and ill-health, with wisdom and strength. This is the fruit of controlling and expanding the life-force energy called *prana.* Powerful, simple and beneficial practices which utilize the life-force in the breath, to rejuvenate the body and transform our emotional, mental and spiritual being.
[208 pages. US$19.5]

Chakra selfHealing by the power of *OM*
Author: *Rudra Shivananda*
A practical workbook on healing and spiritual evolution. Tap into the potential of the primary energy centers of the body, to eliminate depression and fatigue, relieve anxiety and stress, and calm the mind to achieve inner happiness. Learn the effective *yogic* system of tuning, balancing, color healing, rejuvenation, emotional detoxification, energization, and transcendence, with the *chakras,* in a simple, and step-by-step practice.
[140 pages. US$18.5]

Dew-Drops of the Soul
Author: *Yogiraj Gurunath*
A unique compilation of poetic gems from a contemporary Himalayan Master, expressing the essence of his inner experience, as a guide and inspiration for all spiritual seekers.
[106 pages. US$15.0]

Earth Peace through Self Peace
Author: *Yogiraj Gurunath*
A collection of spiritual talks or *satsangs*, answering the questions from sincere seekers of truth. A Master speaks to the soul through the doorway of the heart, opening the reader to the reality of the true Self, in spite of the limitations of human language. *Yogiraj* speaks from his own direct experience, in his own simple, direct way, clearing away all doubts and irrelevancies.
[164 pages. US$18.5]

Wings to Freedom
Author: *Yogiraj Gurunath Siddhanath*
Mystic Revelations fom the immortal Babaji and other Himalayan Yogis, as experienced by a perfected Master, Yogiraj Gurunath Siddhanath. Follow his footsteps and experience through his words, as he walks his talk in the jungles, temples, ashrams and hidden [to the uninitiated] places of India. Enrich your life with the secret oral traditions revealed for the first time - mysteries of life, immortality and the attainment of Self-Realization.
[308 pages, US$22.5]

Surya Yoga
Author: *Rudra Shivananda*
Tap into the awesome, everpresent healing power of our life-giving Sun. Through the sincere and constant practice of the *Surya Sadhana* [solar practice], you will heal the physical body, acquire greater vitality, overcome all negativity, and also come to a greater understanding and realization of your true nature. Illustrated step-by-step instructions.
[164 pages, US$15.5]

For information on these books or to purchase them on-line with credit card, visit our web-site:
htttp://www.alightbooks.com

www.ingramcontent.com/pod-product-compliance
Lightning Source LLC
Chambersburg PA
CBHW031507270326
41930CB00006B/292